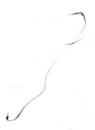

NUTRITIONAL MANAGEMENT OF THE CANCER PATIENT

Nutritional Management of the Cancer Patient

Sponsored by
The University of Texas System
Cancer Center
M. D. Anderson Hospital
and Tumor Institute

Edited by

Joy J. Wollard
Assistant Director of
Clinical Dietetics
The University of Texas
System Cancer Center
M. D. Anderson Hospital
and Tumor Institute
Houston, Texas

Raven Press ▪ New York

Raven Press, 1140 Avenue of the Americas, New York, New York 10036

Made in the United States of America

International Standard Book Number 0–89004–357–4
Library of Congress Catalog Card Number 78–68523

Preface

This volume is intended to provide all those in the health care profession concerned with the care of cancer patients with information that will enable them to better understand the disease, the effects of various treatment modalities, and common complications and the means to resolve them. We examine the metabolic stress of cancer, the interactions between food and drugs received by the cancer patient, and discuss the most significant aspects of nutritional care of the cancer patient from initial nutritional assessment, treatments such as chemotherapy, radiation treatment, and surgery, on through remission and extended care.

Because of the large number of patients treated at The University of Texas System Cancer Center M. D. Anderson Hospital and Tumor Institute, Houston, Texas, the recommendations included in this volume are based on wide experience. We have found that because of the vast number of disease sites and multiple treatment modes no single set of procedures should or could be followed in the care of the cancer patient. There are no simple rules. Each case is unique. What is most important for those involved in the nutritional management of the cancer patient is to never hesitate to be inventive or inquisitive and above all to remember that food intake or lack of it is often the way that patients fight back out of anger, fear, and frustration.

This volume will be of interest to oncologists, surgeons, internists, nutritionists, dietitians, nurses, pharmacists, and all other members of the health care profession concerned with the care of cancer patients.

Joy J. Wollard

Acknowledgments

The introduction written by Dr. van Eys and the chapter on food and drug interactions by Dr. Driever enhance the value of this publication as a complete picture of the nutritional care of the cancer patient. I am grateful for their contributions. I also would like to express my thanks to the dietitians at M. D. Anderson Hospital and Tumor Institute for the many hours spent in preparation of their manuscripts.

Joy J. Wollard

Contents

Contributors

Jeanne Beck, R.D.

Kathleen Bradford, R.D.

Debra Buchanan, R.D.

Patricia Carter, R.D.

Debra S. Dees, R.D.

Carl W. Driever, Ph.D.

Nancy L. Fong, R.D.

Paula K. Hoffman, R.D.

Janice Johnson, M.A., R.D.

Kay Martin, R.D.

Barbara Saunders, R.D.

Debra E. Selig, R.D.

Carol A. Stitt, R.D.

Carolyn Thornton, M.S., R.D.

Jan van Eys, M.D., Ph.D.

Joy J. Wollard, R.D.

The contributors are affiliated with the University of Texas System Cancer Center, M. D. Anderson Hospital and Tumor Institute, Houston, Texas 77030 with the exception of Carl W. Driever, College of Pharmacy, University of Houston, Houston, Texas 77004.

Nutritional Management of the Cancer Patient, edited by J. Wollard.
Raven Press, New York © 1979.

The Metabolic Consequence of Cancer

Jan van Eys

*Department of Pediatrics, The University of Texas System Cancer Center
M. D. Anderson Hospital and Tumor Institute, Houston, Texas 77030*

The clinical association of malnutrition and cancer is known since ancient times. The "Hippocratic Facies" is the classic sign of extreme cancer cachexia. There are obvious reasons why the cancer patient might become malnourished: anorexia, aberrant taste perception, mechanical obstruction of the alimentary tract, malabsorption, nausea, and vomiting; all can contribute. In addition, psychological factors exist: depression, anxiety, and learned association between food and chemotherapy side effects can be major causes of inadequate food intake.

However, the malnutrition in cancer patients can be so extreme that the possibility must be considered that basic metabolic consequences of cancer are ultimate etiological factors. This paper attempts to review some of the systemic effects that malignancy causes, as they pertain to the development of malnutrition.

The consequences of cancer are the result of effects at several levels of integration. First of all, the metabolic peculiarities of the tumor itself. Secondly, the competition of the cancer and host for nutrients, and finally, the distant effects of the cancer on the host.

THE METABOLISM OF THE CANCER CELL

It is very clear from the multitude of diseases that fall under the label cancer that there is not a single "cancer cell" that is common to all tumors. In fact, the classification of tumors is generally on the basis of pathological features that are used to deduce the tissue of origin. It is a dogma in oncology that all cancers have a tissue of origin, and in fact, that it is a specific cell type that has changed into malignant behavior. Therefore, we have leukemias, brain tumors, large bowel cancers, etc. Each, again, in turn has many specialized cells and, therefore, can give rise to many cancers. Leukemias, for instance, can be derived from a number of specific cells in the bone marrow, at various stages of differentiation, resulting in a large number of different leukemias.

Cancers also vary in degree of malignancy. A benign tumor is one that appears microscopically nonaggressive, that does not infiltrate surrounding tissues, and that does not metastasize to distant sites. That does not mean that such tumors cannot kill when they are unfortunately located. Examples of such lethal, yet benign tumors would be tumors in the brain stem, or tumors that affect the heart. Such tumors can affect the nutritional state if there is mechanical obstruction of the bowel or similar direct effects on ordinary physiological functions. However, the metabolism of such benign tumors is not generally different from that found in the normal tissue of origin.

As cancers become more malignant, the cells tend to dedifferentiate: they become gradually less specialized and less recognizable, related to the tissue of origin. In a given cancer, this process may progress with time. While the extremely malignant cell differs still between cancers, the dedifferentiation process tends to continue towards a common metabolic behavior. Therefore, there are metabolic similarities between cancer cells, regardless of the tissue of origin (Table 1).

Much research has been expended on finding a qualitative difference between cancer cells and normal cells. It was hoped that a specific difference would explain malignant behavior. Furthermore, it was hoped that such differences could be exploited therapeutically. There are many quantitative differences, but very few, if any, qualitative differences. The comparison of

TABLE 1. *Metabolic patterns*
of malignant cells

1. Carbohydrate metabolism
    Increased glycolysis
    Decreased gluconeogenesis
    Increased pentone phosphate formation

2. Nucleotide metabolism
    Increased *de novo* purine biosynthesis
    Decreased purine degradation
    Increased pyrimidine biosynthesis
    Decreased pyrimidine degradation
    Increased DNA synthesis

3. Protein and amino acid metabolism
    Increased protein biosynthesis
    Decreased amino acid breakdown
    Decreased urea cycle enzymes

normal and cancer cell metabolism, correlated with the degree of malignancy has recently been reviewed by Weber (25).

One outstanding characteristic of cancer cells is the imbalance between glycolysis and respiration. Glycolysis is the conversion of glucose to lactic acid, while respiration is the oxidation of nutrients, including carbohydrates, to carbon dioxide (1). Glucose is the primary source of energy of cells. Glycolysis and respiration both capture the energy of the substrates as high energy phosphate, primarily in the form of adenosine triphosphate (ATP). However, the efficiency is very different between glycolysis and respiration. One molecule of glucose, when converted to lactic acid (glycolysis) yields two molecules of ATP, while the conversion to carbon dioxide (respiration) could yield as much as 38 molecules of ATP, depending on the completeness of the coupling of oxidative phosphorylation to the electron transport system. Therefore, a respiring tissue can be 19 times as efficient as is a glycolysing tissue in using glucose.

The rate of metabolism is ultimately controlled by the need for energy. This is the general basis for the so-called "Pasteur effect": glycolysis is inhibited by respiration. The molecular mechanism for this effect is an intricate molecular response of glycolytic enzymes to levels of ATP and other phosphate intermediates. However, when ATP is not used, i.e., energy is not needed, metabolism will slow down: glycolysis by the Pasteur effect mechanism, and respiration because there are no adenosine phosphates to convert to ATP. It is possible to demonstrate this metabolic adaptation to need. One can manipulate the energy requirement of the protozoon *Tetrahymena pyriformis* by stopping the cell from swimming. The rate of metabolism adjusts to the energy needs (Table 2) (23).

Cancer cells also have a basic ATP need and adjust their metabolic rate to variations in this need, but they have little or no Pasteur effect. Therefore, relative to normal cells, they squander glucose to achieve the same energy yield. In fact, tumor cells have a strong "Crabtree effect": supplying tumor cells with glucose results in inhibition of endogenous respiration, magnifying the dependence on glucose for energy.

These observations on cancer cells have been extensively tested and repeatedly corroborated. Warburg, who made the original observations, extrapolated these findings into a theory of cancer as damage to respiration (22), but these theories

TABLE 2. *Adjustment of cells to energy needs*

Addition	Respiration relative rate	Glycolysis relative rate
None	1	1
Amytal (5×10^{-4} M)	0.7	8.9
Amytal (2.5×10^{-3} M)	0.05	17.2
Hexamethonium chloride	0.83	0.90

Tetrahymena were tested under oxygen for relative glycolysis and respiration. When an inhibitor of oxidative metabolism was added (the barbiturate amytal) there was a proportionate increase in glycolysis. When the organism was stopped from swimming, i.e., the energy requirement was lowered, respiration decreased significantly but no increase in glycolysis occurred.
Data from ref. 23.

have been vigorously attacked by many, especially Weinhouse (26). They still deserve attention, especially with the new concepts of mitochondria as separate organelles with their own genes (14). The metabolic observations are, however, very germane to the problem of nutrition and cancer, because the host organism must respond to this high demand for glucose by the cancer cell with a high rate of gluconeogenesis from the lactic acid formed by the tumor, the available foodstuff, and nonessential tissue such as muscle. The total tumor burden can be very high; when tumor glycolysis overwhelms the host, lactic acidosis can occur in leukemia as a very serious complication (4). The situation is aggravated by the frequent anaerobic condition inside poorly vascularized solid tumors.

This high demand on gluconeogenesis will result in a severe catabolic state. Actual increases in caloric demand in extensive cancers have not always been documented, though a few studies are suggestive of a reduced efficiency of energy utilization (27). The extreme cases, where the tumor burden is very great, usually show an increased need for calories above the ability of the host to ingest. When the availability of glucose is limited, the tumor can compete successfully with the host. Normal cells usually have no Crabtree effect and maintain respiration from other nutrient sources even when glucose is supplied. Therefore, the cancer cell utilizes the glucose preferentially. Comparison of the glucose uptake by tumor and host showed an almost complete removal of interstitial fluid glucose by the tumor while the normal tissue extracted only one-third of the available glucose, as judged from the circulatory blood level (12).

Such calculations of glucose utilization and equation to ATP yield must be taken with some reservation. Many reactions occur in tissues that squander energy for the generation of heat (16). It is conceivable that the excessive wastage of energy in such cycles is the major cause of the excess glucose consumption. However, there is no evidence as yet that tumor tissues have more or more active "futile" metabolic cycles than normal tissues.

THE COMPETITION OF TUMOR AND HOST
FOR NUTRIENTS

Just as there is no single tumor cell, there is no single metabolic consequence of cancer on the host. However, as the cancer bulk increases and the malignancy is more advanced, common consequences tend to become visible, with as extreme consequence, cancer cachexia.

A primary consequence of extensive cancer is gluconeogenesis. There is active utilization of amino acids for this purpose, especially alanine. If food intake is inadequate, endogenous nitrogen sources, such as muscle protein, are used. This is not unique to cancer patients. Protein is used for gluconeogenesis during any period of protein-energy malnutrition (2). The extreme demand on glucose can accelerate the process significantly. However, in addition, there is some suggestive evidence that the cancer-bearing host does not always respond normally to starvation (6). Normal individuals attempt to adapt to chronic starvation by change of the body from glucose to ketone bodies as a utilizable fuel. Glucose formation still continues but both heart and brain will utilize ketone bodies (17). The primary fuel for survival changes from protein derived glucose, to fat. Whenever there is a major insult, such adaptation might be impaired. When the cancer is extensive, there may be similar impairment. From experience with total parenteral nutrition in tumor-bearing hosts, Brennan has suggested an aggravated nitrogen and caloric requirement to stay in weight balance even though the basic metabolic rate was not elevated in such patients (6). Others actually do find an increase in the basic metabolic rate of patients with cancer and believe that is one of the reasons for the development of cancer cachexia (24).

Caloric restriction is often cited as inhibitory to tumor growth. Therefore, it is argued, feeding the host is counterproductive and feeds the tumor as well (7). However, once a cancer is established, the tumor competes effectively with the host. Even if absolute tumor weight might be diminished, tumor weight

TABLE 3. *Neuroblastoma patients stage IV*

Nutrition during treatment	Initial status	Outcome
Intravenous hyperalimentation	Well nourished	3/3 remained well nourished
	Malnourished	3/3 became well nourished
No intravenous hyperalimentation	Well nourished	2/5 became malnourished

All patients were treated by intensive protocol. Of the patients not on hyperalimentation, three were made well nourished by prior intravenous hyperalimentation but were not so fed during the chemotherapy.
Data from ref. 20.

relative to body weight will be high, as is the obvious experience in all patients with active cancer who die of cachexia. Conversely, feeding of animals with active tumor did not stimulate the tumor out of proportion to the host (8). Thus, while the tumor competes effectively in circumstances of limited nutrient availability, tumors are not capable of inhibiting normal body growth and homeostasis. Even young children with advanced neuroblastoma can be restored to nutritional adequacy by parenteral hyperalimentation (Table 3) (20).

DISTAL EFFECTS OF TUMORS

It would be attractive to speculate that tumors excrete a "toxo-hormone," a substance effective distally to interfere with the basic metabolism of the host to account for the significant changes found. It is almost impossible to prove that something does *not* exist. However, it is unnecessary to postulate such a mechanism. In general the degree of problems the host experiences is a function of the tumor size. In man, tumor size may reach up to 5% of total body weight, but generally is much lower. The extreme metabolic derangements described in animals often had models where the tumor weight exceeded 30% of the total body weight.

The component of anorexia in cancer is very real. It is clearly a major factor in weight loss in many patients. While tumor toxins are a possible etiology it is more likely that psychological factors play a major part. Furthermore, lactic acid could be that tumor toxin (3). The possible causes of anorexia have been briefly reviewed, but in the context of metabolic disorders as another major cause of the weight loss (9).

The major instance where distal effects of tumors are seen occurs when the tumors secrete hormones themselves. Such ectopic hormone secretion has been described for a variety of tumors and with a variety of hormones. These hormones can be metabolically active, as far as we know. Erythropoietin excretion by hypernephromas and hepatomas is well known (15). Adrenocorticotropic hormone secretion is well documented, especially by bronchogenic carcinomas (18). A number of tumors generate hormone-like substances that would be expected to be produced by their tissue of origin, but which are now made in uncontrolled amounts. The classic examples are the neural crest tumors, neuroblastomas and pheochromocytomas which make catecholamines (21), and intestinal neoplasms, the Zollinger Ellison syndrome and other multiple endocrine adenomatoses which make gastrointestinal hormones (13). These tumors can have profound effects on the patient's metabolic and nutritional state.

The hyperglycemia also found in patients with malignancy has suggested that there might be frequent hyperinsulin secretion. The hyperlactacidemia could actually stimulate gluconeogenesis (11). When a large number of patients with cancer were evaluated by glucose tolerance tests, 37% of cancer patients and 9% of patients with benign disease had abnormal tests (10). Those patients with abnormal results were all older, i.e., above 30 years of age. However, such a high incidence of abnormal glucose homeostasis is not corroborated by others. Certainly insulin levels are said to be appropriate for blood glucose levels (5).

Thus, while many hormonally mediated paraneoplastic syndromes exist, it is reasonable to assert that the distant effects of the tumor all relate to its abnormal metabolism and are proportional to its bulk.

EXTREME MALNUTRITION AND CANCER CACHEXIA

The extreme form of malnutrition seen in the cancer patient is cachexia. It is often described as a special syndrome. Many of the metabolic consequences of cancer are thought to contribute to this extreme state of catabolism. However, no real, specific view of cachexia needs to be taken. There is no need to generate a specific hypothesis of its development (19). The contribution of inadequate intake, extra caloric demands by the tumor, coupled with frequent, vigorous therapy can usually explain this classic outcome of the disease.

It is more important to remember that malnutrition has a high mortality when it reaches that extreme a state. The possibility of metabolic derangements from malnutrition alone, as well as the extreme susceptibility to infection, makes rehabilitation of the extremely malnourished patient a medical challenge. It is a slow process at best, and therefore must be prevented rather than cured.

REFERENCES

1. Aisenberg, A. C. (1960): *The Glycolysis and Respiration of Tumors.* Academic Press, New York.
2. Alleyne, G. A. O., Hay, R. W., Picou, D. I., Stanfield, J. P., and Whitehead, R. G. (1977): *Protein Energy Malnutrition.* Edward Arnold Publishers, Ltd., London.
3. Baile, C. A., Zinn, W. M., and Mayer, L. (1970): Effects of lactate and other metabolites on food intakes of monkeys. *Am. J. Physiol.,* 219:1606–1613.
4. Blocke, J. B. (1974): Lactic acidosis in malignancy and observations on its possible pathogenesis. *Ann. N.Y. Acad. Sci.,* 230:94–102.
5. Brennan, M. F. (1978): Host versus tumor metabolism. *The Cancer Bulletin,* 30:72–77.
6. Brennan, M. F. (1977): Uncomplicated starvation versus cancer cachexia. *Cancer Res.,* 37:2359–2364.

7. Clayson, D. B. (1975): Nutrition and experimental carcinogenesis: A review. *Cancer Res.,* 35:3292–3300.
8. Copeland, E. M., Daly, J. M., Guin, E., et al. (1976): Effects of synthetic amino acids on cell-mediated immunity. *Surgical Forum,* 27:113–114.
9. Costa, C. (1977): Cachexia, the metabolic component of neoplastic disease. *Cancer Res.,* 37:2321–2335.
10. Glicksman, A. S., and Rawson, R. W. (1956): Diabetes and altered carbohydrate metabolism in patients with cancer. *Cancer,* 9:1127–1134.
11. Gold, J. (1974): Cancer cachexia and gluconeogenesis. *Ann. N.Y. Acad. Sci.,* 230:103–110.
12. Gullino, P., Grantham, F. H., Courtney, A. H., et al. (1967): Relationship between oxygen and glucose consumption by transplanted tumors *in vivo, Cancer Res.,* 27:1041–1052.
13. Haverbache, B. J., and Dyce, B. J. (1974): Gastrin, multiple and endocrine adenomatosis, and the Zollinger Ellison syndrome. *Ann. N.Y. Acad. Sci.,* 230:297–305.
14. Hoberman, H. D. (1975): Is there a role for mitochondrial genes in carcinogenesis. *Cancer Res.,* 35:3332–3335.
15. Krantz, S. B., and Jacobson, L. O. (1970): *Erythropoietin and the Regulation of Erythropoiesis.* University of Chicago Press, Chicago.
16. Newsholme, E. A. (1976): Substrate cycles in metabolic regulation and heat generation. *Biochem. Soc. Symp.,* 41:61–109.
17. Owen, O. E., Morgan, A. P., Kemp, H. G., Sullivan, L. M., Herrera, M. G., and Caholl, G. F., Jr. (1967): Brain metabolism during fasting. *J. Clin. Invest.* 46:1589–1595.
18. Omenn, G. J., and Wilkins, E. W. (1974): Hormone syndromes associated with bronchogenic carcinoma. *J. Thoracic Cardiovascular Surg.* 59:877–881.
19. Theologides, A. (1974): The anorexia-cachexia syndrome: A new hypothesis. *Ann. N.Y. Acad. Sci.,* 230:14–22.
20. van Eys, J.: Malnutrition in children with cancer—incidence and consequence. *Cancer (in press).*
21. Voorhess, M. L. (1974): Neuroblastoma—pheochromocytoma: Products and pathogenesis. *Ann. N.Y. Acad. Sci.,* 230:187–194.
22. Warburg, O. M. (1962): *New Methods of Cell Physiology, Applied to Cancer, Photosynthesis, and Mechanism of X-ray Section,* pp. 322–334 and 627–632. Interscience Publishers, New York.
23. Warnock, L. G., and van Eys, J. (1963): Energy expenditure and metabolic regulation in *Tetrahymena pyriformis. J. Cell. Comp. Physiol.,* 61:309.
24. Warnold, J., Lundholm, J., and Schersten, T. (1978): Energy balance and body composition in cancer patients. *Cancer Res.,* 38:1801–1807.
25. Weber, G. (1977): Enzymology of cancer cells. *N. Engl. J. Med.,* 296:486–493.

26. Weinhouse, S. (1960): Enzyme activities and tumor progression. In: *Amino Acids, Proteins and Cancer Biochemistry* edited by J. T. Edsall, pp. 109–119. Academic Press, New York.
27. Young, V. (1977): Energy metabolism and requirements in the cancer patient. *Cancer Res.*, 37:2336–2347.

Nutritional Management of the Cancer Patient, edited by J. Wollard.
Raven Press, New York © 1979.

Food and Drug Interactions in the Cancer Patient

Carl W. Driever

*Department of Clinical Pharmacy, University of Houston College of Pharmacy,
Houston, Texas 77004*

The overall topic of drug interactions is a very complex one involving many different specific types of drug interactions (Table 1). For purposes of this chapter, I will deal primarily with drug and food interactions. There are numerous reports in the literature on the subject of the interrelationships between drugs and various foods (1,4–6,11). This discussion will be limited primarily to the following: (a) A review of the mechanisms responsible for the occurrence of food and drug interactions, and (b) A summary of information on some of the most significant interrelationships between diet and drug therapy, particularly chemotherapy.

Before examining specific mechanisms and specific interactions, it would be useful to review what happens to a drug when it is administered to a patient (Fig. 1). With a few exceptions (e.g., intravenous or intraarterial drug administraton) drugs must first be *absorbed* into the circulatory system from the site of administration. This involves the passage of the drug molecule across biological membranes, generally by passive diffusion, but there are examples of active transport mechanisms as well. Once absorption has taken place, drugs exist in either the "free form" or the so-called "bound form." At this point, it is important to remember that it is the amount of the "free form" at any given moment that is responsible for the ultimate activity of the drug. The main plasma component to which drugs can be reversibly bound is albumin; however, drugs can bind to other proteins

TABLE 1. *Types of drug interactions*

1. Drug-drug interactions
2. Drug-chemical interactions
3. Drug-body substrate interactions
4. Drug-disease interactions
5. Drug interactions caused by genetic influences
6. Drug interactions caused by residual drug effects
7. Drug resistance

and other constituents of the plasma as well. Drugs can be further *distributed* to other parts of the body where they exert their action or are stored, possibly in another bound form. After distribution, drugs can be 'stored' in a number of body compartments (protein, water, fat, etc.). Drugs can either be *excreted* unchanged by the kidney or distributed to the liver where they are *metabolized,* generally to inactive metabolites which can then be diffused back into the plasma and be excreted by the kidneys. Drug metabolism is sometimes equated to inactivation of drugs. In most cases this is valid; however,

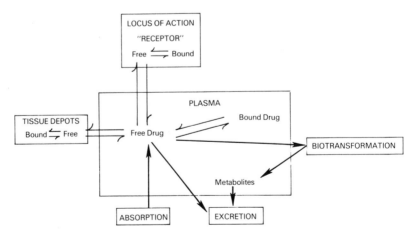

FIG. 1. Schematic diagram of drug disposition. (From ref. 3, with permission.)

there are some instances where metabolism can result in the formation of a more active and sometimes a more toxic compound than the parent compound. These are referred to as active metabolites. A great number of drug interactions, in general, and food and drug interactions, in particular, can occur as a result of interference (increase or decrease) with absorption, distribution, metabolism, excretion, or combinations of these phenomena.

DRUG INTERFERENCE WITH NUTRITIONAL STATUS

The various mechanisms by which drugs can interfere with the nutritional status of a patient are shown in Table 2. Some of the drug categories which can cause this interference are shown in Table 3. Many of these drugs are used in the treatment of chronic conditions, thereby posing a threat to patients' nutritional status. Of those drug categories listed, the most significant ones for cancer patients include: anticonvulsants (8,9), antimicrobials (2,7), corticosteroids (3), and cytotoxic agents (10). Results of the various interferences may range from appetite suppression (e.g., azathioprine, bleomycin, etc.) to a number of different malabsorption syndromes and vitamin and

TABLE 2. *Mechanisms by which drugs can interfere with nutritional status*

Appetite changes (suppression or stimulation)
Changes in nutrient absorption
    Changes in gastrointestinal transit time
    Changes in gastrointestinal pH
    Changes in bile acid activity
    Changes in peristalsis
    Changes in absorptive enzymes
    Changes in cell structure of gastrointestinal tract
    Complexation
Changes in nutrient's metabolism and utilization
Changes in nutrient's excretion

From ref. 6.

TABLE 3. *Drug categories caus-ing interference with nutritional status*

Antacids
Anorexients
Anticonvulsants
Antidepressants
Antimicrobials
Appetite stimulants
Autonomic agents
   Anticholinergics
   Ganglionic blockers
Cathartics-laxatives
Corticosteroids
Cytotoxic drugs (folic acid antagonists)
Diuretics
Hypocholesterolemic agents
Oral contraceptives
Surfactants

From ref. 6.

other nutrient deficiencies (e.g., methotrexate, antibiotics, etc.). Probably the most significant of the interactions between foods and drugs in cancer patients, from the standpoint of frequency, is the nausea and vomiting associated with the vast majority of chemotherapeutic agents. For this reason, hyperalimentation must sometimes be employed.

DIETARY INTERFERENCE WITH DRUG THERAPY

Just as drugs may adversely influence a patient's nutritional status, various dietary components as well as dietary patterns may interact with the drug therapy of a particular patient. The various mechanisms by which diet can interfere with drug therapy are shown in Table 4. Note that the mechanisms are very similar to those discussed above. Circumstances may often exist that warrant concurrent food intake with drugs. Some drugs that are used in cancer patients are very irritating when taken on an empty stomach and thus should be taken immediately

TABLE 4. *Mechanisms by which foods can interfere with drug therapy*

Changes in absorption of orally administered drugs
   Change in gastrointestinal transit time and motility
   Change in gastrointestinal secretions and pH
   Change in osmolality of gastrointestinal tract
   Change in ionization of drug
   Change in stability of drug
   Change in solubility of drug
   Complexation of drug by dietary component
Change in drug's distribution
Change in drug's metabolism
Change in drug's excretion
Agonistic or antagonistic pharmacologic response by active substance in food

From ref. 6.

after meals, or with food or milk, and include: chlorpromazine, ferrous salts, steroids (hydrocortisone, prednisolone, prednisone), and potassium supplements (11). The presence of food with these agents may reduce their irritating effects. On the other hand, circumstances also exist that preclude ingesting certain foods with drugs. Some examples of drugs that should be taken on an empty stomach include: ampicillin, cloxacillin, dipyridamole, erythromycin base, lincomycin, penicillin G potassium, and tetracycline (11). The significance of the particular interference is dependent upon *both* the drug and the condition being treated.

Perhaps some of the most dangerous interactions of dietary components with drugs are those resulting from the action of a food constituent. Some pharmacologically active constituents are glycyrrhizinic acid (licorice), oxalates, potassium, and tyramine. The combination of tyramine and certain drugs can be a lethal one. When ingested, tyramine can cause a massive release of norepinephrine and epinephrine from postganglionic sympathetic neurons and the adrenal medulla. Epinephrine and norephrine (and other sympathomimetic amines) can cause vasoconstriction and increased heart rate. Under normal circumstances this is harmless, but in the presence of certain drugs (particularly

TABLE 5. *Foods contain-
ing tyramine*[a]

1. Cheese
    A. Camembert
    B. Emmentaler
    C. Cheddar
    D. Gruyere
    E. Processed American
2. Pickled herring
3. Chicken livers
4. Yogurt
5. Yeast products
6. Broad beans
7. Canned figs
8. Chocolate
9. Alcoholic beverages
    A. Wine (Chianti, Sherry)
    B. Beer
10. Coffee

[a] *Reactions with the above*
may result in headaches hy-
pertension, cardiac arrhyth-
mias, intracranial bleeding,
circulatory failure, and possibly death.

monoamine oxidase inhibitors), it can result in serious problems.
Monoamine oxidase is an enzyme that normally breaks down
catecholamines such as norepinephrine and epinephrine to inactive metabolites. If this enzyme is inhibited, these agents can
exert their effects much longer than otherwise possible. The
best known examples of monoamine oxidase inhibitors are
pargyline (Eutonyl®), phenelzine (Nardil®), and isocarboxazid
(Marplan®). There are a few other agents that, in addition to
their primary effects, also inhibit monoamine oxidase as a side
effect. Procarbazine (Matulane®) is in this group of drugs and
is mentioned because of its use in the treatment of neoplastic
disease, particularly Hodgkin's disease. Table 5 lists some of the
more common foods that contain significant amounts of tyramine

and can pose a threat to patients who are taking one of the monoamine oxidase inhibitors.

REFERENCES

1. American Pharmaceutical Association (1976): *Evaluations of Drug Interactions,* Second Edition, American Pharmaceutical Association, Washington, D.C.
2. Eanes, R. Z. (1962): Diet in relation to antimicrobial therapy. *Pediatr. Clin. North. Am.,* 9:1033.
3. Goodman, L. S., and Gilman, A. (1975): *The Pharmacological Basis of Therapeutics,* Fifth Edition, pp. 1477–1503. MacMillan Publishing Co., New York.
4. Hansten, P. (1975): *Drug Interactions,* Third Edition. Lea and Febiger, Philadelphia.
5. Hartshorn, E. A. (1977): Food and drug interactions. *Guidelines to Professional Pharmacy,* 4 (3):1.
6. Hethcox, J. M., and Stanaszek, W. F. (1974): Interactions of drugs and diet. *Hosp. Pharm.,* 9:373.
7. Kunin, C. M., and Finland, M. (1971): Clinical pharmacology of the tetracycline antibiotics. *Clin. Pharm. Ther.,* 2:51.
8. Reynolds, E. H., et al. (1968): Reversible absorption defects in anticonvulsant megaloblastic anemia. *J. Clin. Pathol.,* 18:593.
9. Richens, A., and Row, D. J. (1970): Disturbance of calcium metabolism by anticonvulsant drugs. *Br. Med. J.,* 4:73.
10. Roe, D. A. (1973): Nutritional side effects of drugs. *Foods and Nutrition News,* 45:1.
11. Shore, M. F. (1971): A time for drugs. *Can. Pharm. J.,* 104:99–108.

Nutritional Management of the Cancer Patient, edited by J. Wollard.
Raven Press, New York © 1979.

Nutritional Assessment of the Adult Cancer Patient

Jeanne Beck

Research Dietetic Services, Cancer Clinical Research Center, University of Texas System Cancer Center M. D. Anderson Hospital and Tumor Institute, Houston, Texas 77030

Nutritional assessment is the first step in the prevention and treatment of malnutrition (4). Since 1975, when formalized nutritional assessment was first suggested as a necessary factor in preventing hospital malnutrition by Butterworth and Blackburn (7), it has been gaining importance in both medical and dietetic fields.

Nutritional assessment is the systematic evaluation of a patient's current state of nutrition, using both physical and biochemical means. The assessment includes three major parameters: nutrition history, anthropometrics, and laboratory analysis (4,5,7,8). The assessment must consider as many parameters as possible because, at present, no single test can determine nutritional status (5,7,9,11,25,31). The greater the number of parameters used, the more conclusive the assessment will be (5,7,9,11,25,31).

A nutritional assessment of the cancer patient is no different from nutritional assessment of other patients. However, in interpreting some laboratory test results, we need to consider that neoplastic disease and its treatments can alter the nutritional significance of the test (6,10,11,24).

NUTRITION HISTORY PARAMETERS

The first parameter to include in the nutritional assessment is the patient's nutrition history. This includes a thorough diet his-

FIGURE 1.

INITIAL NUTRITION HISTORY

Date:	Day of Study:	Name:	Pt. No.
Study No.	Randomization:	Address:	Phone:
Physician:		Birthdate:	Age:	Sex:
Diagnosis:		Occupation:	
		Present Employment Status:	
Therapy Dates:		Living Conditions During Study:	
Treatment Protocol:		Present Diet:	Past Diet:
Pertinent Facts from Medical Record:		Medications Presently Taking:	

RECENT GAIN OR LOSS IN WEIGHT	% Loss or Gain	FACTORS CONTRIBUTING TO WEIGHT LOSS OR GAIN
1 month		G.I. Disturbances
		Nausea and/or Vomiting

3 month

6 month

Comments:

Diarrhea

Other

Mouth Soreness and/or Swallowing Difficulties

Change in Appetite

Change in Sense of Smell or Taste

Food Likes and Dislikes

Pain and/or Breathing Difficulties

Height _____ Present Wt. _____ Usual Wt. _____
(w/o shoes)   (w/o shoes)

Wrist _____ Body Frame _____ Desirable
Measurement   Type   Wt. _____

RDA for Present Wt. _____ RDA for Usual Wt. _____

Kcal. _____ PRO _____ Kcal. _____ PRO _____

ANTHROPOMETRIC MEASUREMENTS	% Standard
Upper Arm Length (left)	
Midpoint	
Arm Circumference (left)	
Triceps Skin Fold	
Arm Muscle Circumference	
Ideal Creatinine for Height	

Urea(0785) _____ Urinary(0842) _____
Nitrogen   Creatinine
Creatinine/ _____ Nitrogen _____
Ht. Index   Balance
(0241)   (0891)
Albumin _____ T.I.B.C. _____
Serum Transferrin(0.8 × TIBC)-43 _____
(0823) _____ (0858)
B-12 _____ C(0106) _____ Folic _____
(0131)   (0311)
Carotene _____ T. Lymph Count _____

FIGURE 2.

NUTRITIONAL FOLLOW-UP

Name: _____   Time Spent: _____

Date: _____   Weight: _____
                      (w/o shoes)

Day of Study: _____

ANTHROPOMETRIC MEASURES   % Standard

Arm Circumference _____

Triceps Skin Fold _____

Arm Muscle Circumference _____

LAB DATA

Nitrogen Balance _____
Creatinine/Ht. Index _____
Urinary(0842) _____   Ideal Creatinine
Creatinine _____   for Ht. _____
Urea(0785) _____ (0891)
Nitrogen _____   T.I.B.C. _____
Serum Transferrin(0.8 × TIBC)-43 _____
(0823) _____   (0858)
B-12 _____   C(0106) _____   Folic _____
(0131) _____   (0311) _____
Carotene _____   T. Lymph Count _____
Albumin(0241) _____

FACTORS CONTRIBUTING TO WEIGHT LOSS OR GAIN

G.I. Disturbances
Nausea and/or Vomiting

Diarrhea

Other

Mouth Soreness and/or Swallowing Difficulties

Change in Appetite

Change in Sense of Smell or Taste

Food Likes and Dislikes

Pain and/or Breathing Difficulties

Food Intakes Given:

24 HOUR RECALL

Meal Period	Food	Amount	CHO	PRO	FAT	KCAL
Morning						
Mid AM						
Noon						
Mid PM						
Evening						
PM						
TOTALS						

FIGURE 3.

24 HOUR RECALL

Date: _____

Meal Period	Food	Amount	CHO	PRO	FAT	KCAL
Morning						
Mid AM						
Noon						
Mid PM						
Evening						
PM						
TOTALS						

Comments on Recall:

Comments on Instruction: _____ Time Spent: _____

Materials given to patient:

Food Intake Records Given to Patient:

tory and interview with the patient, preferably with his family in attendance, and a review of the medical record (Figs. 1 and 2).

Diet History and Interview

The diet history and interview should cover dietary patterns prior to illness and during any past treatments. Questions such as usual weight prior to illness and recent weight changes, changes in sense of taste or smell related to food and to past treatments, and changes in appetite and food likes and dislikes related to the onset of disease and to previous treatments should be included in the interview.

A 24-hr dietary recall (Fig. 3) is important in assessing current dietary patterns and intake. The 24-hr dietary recall has its limitations (1,8,22,29), but it is a useful tool when used in the proper perspective.

The diet history and interview are important not only in assessing nutritional status, but also in developing the nutritional care plan. The diet history and interview help the dietitian to assess both the patient's physical and mental capabilities for following a nutritional care plan and the type of instruction and reinforcement the patient and his family will need.

Medical Record Review

The review of the medical record (Fig. 1) should include the present state of the patient's disease, the location of the disease, past treatments and responses to those treatments, past weights, and proposed treatment plans. The medical record review gives the dietitian a more in-depth view of the patient's capabilities for following a nutritional care plan and aids in indicating possible problem areas.

ANTHROPOMETRIC PARAMETERS

The second parameter to include in the nutritional assessment is the anthropometric measurement of nutritional status. The current anthropometric measurements are considered rough measurements (11), but when used in conjunction with the biochemical tests, they represent an effective practical tool for assessing nutritional status and the effects of nutritional support (11).

The anthropometric parameters include weight, height, and wrist measurement to determine body frame type and ideal body weight; triceps skin fold thickness; and arm muscle circumference. Other anthropometric parameters, such as subscapular skin fold, may also be used. Based on a careful research of the anthropometric parameters available for assessing nutritional status, each nutritional support service must determine which measurements and which methods best meet its own patient needs. Blackburn and Bistrian (4) make recommendations about frequency of reassessment, but each nutritional unit must decide for itself how often to repeat the measurements, as determined by its own patient population and the type of nutritional support used. It is important to standardize both the measurements and the frequence of repeating them, since standardization of procedures aids in accurately evaluating the success or failure of the nutritional care plan (11).

Height and Weight

An accurate measurement of height and weight is important in evaluating the patient's present weight loss or weight gain, and in determining the ideal body weight for height (4,5,7). The body frame type can be determined by taking a wrist measurement on the nondominant arm distal to the styloid process of the radius and ulna (Fig. 4), and comparing this measurement to a chart for determining body frame size (20). An accurate determination of body frame size is helpful in estimating ideal body weight.

Triceps Skin Fold

The measurement of the triceps skin fold thickness indicates the patient's available fat reserve (17). The triceps skin fold

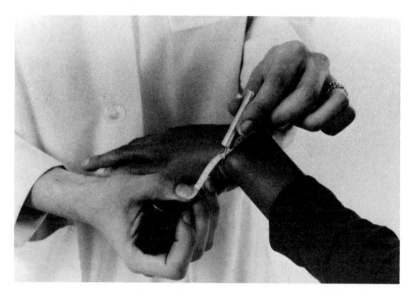

FIG. 4. Wrist measurement.

is preferred over the subscapular skin fold because it is easily accessible to both patient and examiner (4,9), it is presumed to be less involved in subclinical edema (9), and it has shown greater reliability over the subscapular skin fold in assessing obesity (26). The triceps skin fold has one disadvantage, however: it may yield a falsely low measure if the skin and subcutaneous fat are being stretched by underlying muscle hypertrophy (17). The subscapular skin fold has the advantage of providing a uniform layer of subcutaneous fat and the disadvantage of inaccessibility (17).

The technique for determining the triceps skin fold (17) begins with finding the midpoint of the arm between the acromial process of the scapula and the olecranon process of the elbow (Fig. 5). The nondominant arm or the left arm should be used for this measurement. The tables currently used for comparing triceps skin fold and arm muscle circumference data are based upon using the left arm measurement only (17), not the nondominant arm, which can be either the left or right arm.

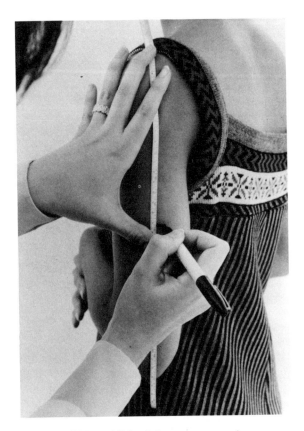

FIG. 5. Midpoint measurement.

The purpose for selecting the left or nondominant arm is to prevent a false-positive measure due to the greater degree of muscle development present in the dominant arm. The important point to remember is to standardize procedures; either always use the left arm or always use the nondominant arm.

The triceps skin fold measurement (17,18) is taken on the back of the arm at the previously determined midpoint by pinching the skin parallel to the body (Fig. 6). The pinch pulls the layer of fat and skin away from the underlying muscle. The calipers for measuring the skin fold thickness are placed on the

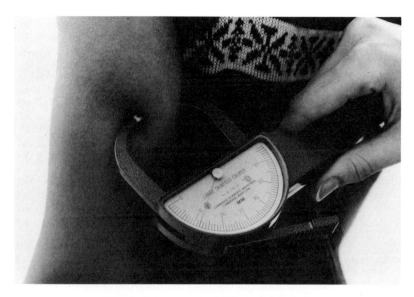

FIG. 6. Triceps skin fold measurement.

pinch. The pinch is released for three seconds and the measurement is read from the dial on the calipers. It is important to use accurate calipers, such as the Harpenden or Lange calipers.

The skin fold is measured three times, with the average reading of the three becoming the triceps skin fold measurement used for comparison with the table of standards, Table 1 (17). The standards for adult triceps skin fold were developed using

TABLE 1. *Table of standards, triceps skin fold—adults*[a]

	Triceps skin fold (mm)				
Sex	100% of standard	90% of standard	80% of standard	70% of standard	60% of standard
Male	12.5	11.3	10.0	8.8	7.5
Female	16.5	14.9	13.2	11.6	9.0

Example: TSF = (6.0 + 6.5 + 6.5)/3 = 6.3 mm = 38% of standard (female).

[a] Adapted from ref. 17.

international measurements (17); new tables are presently being developed for the United States population (16).

It is important to standardize the technique used by the nutrition support team for measuring the triceps skin fold. Accurate interpretation of the percent standard for the triceps skin fold is also important, since some persons have a normally small layer of fat at the triceps, yet are considered well nourished. The triceps skin fold is just one of many parameters to be used in determining nutritional status. The first triceps skin fold measurement should also be used as a base line, allowing comparison as the patient is monitored.

Arm Muscle Circumference

The mid-upper-arm muscle circumference is an indicator of lean body mass or muscle tissue (4,17). If a patient is malnourished, he will have not only diminished fat stores, but also decreased lean body mass (4,7).

To determine the mid-upper-arm muscle circumference, the circumference of the arm is taken at the previously determined midpoint (Fig. 7) using a nonstretchable metal tape measure (17). To find the arm muscle circumference (AMC), a formula developed by Jelliffe (17) and adapted by Blackburn (4) must be used (Fig. 8). The arm muscle circumference is equal to the arm circumference minus the triceps skin fold multiplied by π (3.14) (17). The purpose for multiplying the triceps skin fold by π, then subtracting this figure from the arm circumference, is to take into account the layer of skin and fat that surrounds the arm muscle (17).

The arm muscle circumference is compared to a standard, Table 2, developed by Jelliffe (17). These standards are also based on international measurements (17), and standards for the United States are currently being developed (16).

Accurate interpretation of the percent standard for the arm muscle circumference is also important. Some persons may normally have underdeveloped arm muscles yet be considered

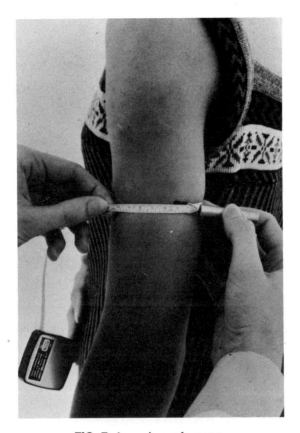

FIG. 7. Arm circumference.

well nourished, or they may have overdeveloped arm muscles resulting from manual labor or exercise and be considered malnourished. The arm muscle circumference is only one of many parameters used to assess nutritional status, and should be used as a baseline figure for future comparison as well as an assessment tool.

The arm muscle circumference may be altered if the muscle is swollen from a recent injection into the arm. In this case the measurement should be repeated in a few days or the opposite arm should be used. All difficulties encountered or changes in

$$\begin{array}{l} \text{Arm} \\ \text{circumference} - \\ \text{(AC)} \\ \text{in centimeters} \end{array} \left[\begin{array}{c} \text{Triceps} \\ 3.14\ (\pi) \times \text{skin fold} \\ \text{(TSF)} \\ \text{in grams} \end{array} \right] = \begin{array}{l} \text{Arm} \\ \text{muscle} \\ \text{circumference} \\ \text{in centimeters} \end{array}$$

Example: 10.0 − (3.14 × 0.60) = AMC
10.0 − (1.88) = AMC
8.12 cm = AMC

FIG. 8. Formula for calculating arm muscle circumference. (Adapted from refs. 5 and 17.)

TABLE 2. *Table of standards, arm muscle circumference—adults*[a]

Sex	Arm muscle circumference (cm)				
	100% of standard	90% of standard	80% of standard	70% of standard	60% of standard
Male	29.3	26.3	23.4	20.5	17.6
Female	28.5	25.7	22.8	20.0	17.1

Example: AMC = 9.92 cm = 35% of standard (female).
[a] Adapted from ref. 17.

procedure should be noted and dated on the nutritional assessment form.

LABORATORY PARAMETERS

The third parameter to include in the nutritional assessment is the laboratory measurement of nutritional status. Numerous tests are available for assessing vitamin and mineral deficiencies (8,25), as are detailed clinical descriptions of these deficiencies (8,17). This chapter, therefore, will not discuss vitamin and mineral deficiencies but will focus on protein status and some of the laboratory tests currently used to assess it.

Visceral Protein Status

Serum albumin and serum transferrin, or total iron binding capacity, are used as indicators of visceral protein status (2,4,

5). Serum albumin may be lowered for several reasons, such as increased losses in renal or gastrointestinal disease or reduced synthesis caused by liver disease (4). It is usually decreased in malnutrition (2,4,7,17) and hypoalbuminemia occurs frequently in cancer patients (10). The hypoalbuminemia present in cancer patients may be due to depressed synthesis of albumin, which is possibly a manifestation of the systemic effects of cancer (11). Serum transferrin, or total iron binding capacity, is considered a more sensitive indicator of visceral protein status than serum albumin (4). Serum transferrin is the protein in the blood that transports iron, and the iron binding capacity (TIBC) represents the total amount of iron that can be carried in the plasma by transferrin (12). Laboratory values for serum transferrin or total iron binding capacity are abnormally low in protein-calorie malnutrition, and increase as nutritional status improves (2,4).

The hematology profile also is a component of the nutritional assessment (4,8,17). A reduced lymphocyte count is associated with malnutrition (2,4,7,17), as well as with other anemias (7,17). The interpretation of the hematology profile in the cancer patient merits special attention. Various kinds of anemias are present in most advanced cancer and leukemia patients, and some chemotherapeutic agents also cause various anemias (18). The anemia associated with chemotherapy may be different from the anemia associated with malnutrition (23); therefore, the effect of adequate nutrition upon this type of anemia is not known.

Nitrogen Balance

A simplified formula for assessing nitrogen balance has been developed to evaluate protein utilization in humans (4,5,21). This simplified formula is a useful tool, but persons utilizing it should be aware that it is controversial. The resulting simplified nitrogen balance should not be considered a sensitive assessment (6,10,11,14). Sources of error exist both in the method of collecting data to calculate the formula and in the possibilities of unmeasured losses (10,11,14). Controversies concern the period of time the urine collections should last, the best method to obtain the dietary intake during urine collections, the effect dietary intake prior to the urine collection has on the nitrogen excreted, and accounting for errors in the collection of urine samples (10,11,14). Evidence suggests the existence of a pathway for nitrogen losses that is so far unmeasured (11). In addition, the effect of tumor growth upon nitrogen retention is poorly understood (6,10,11). All of these factors decrease the significance of the simplified nitrogen balance for the cancer patient.

The formula used to calculate nitrogen balance (Fig. 9) requires a 24-hr urine collection to determine the total urea nitrogen excreted in a 24-hr period. During this same 24-hr period the patient's dietary intake must be recorded. It is preferable to have dietary intakes for both the 24 hr before the urine collection and for the 24 hr during the collection, and to average these to obtain the nitrogen intake used in the formula.

The nitrogen balance is simply the oral nitrogen intake minus the urinary nitrogen losses plus a constant for nitrogen losses from non-urea urinary nitrogen compounds, feces, skin, hair, and nails. The constant used in the formula for calculating simplified nitrogen balance varies in the sources reviewed. The constant

$$\frac{\text{Nitrogen}}{\text{balance}} = \frac{\text{Grams protein from oral intake}/24 \text{ hr}}{6.25 \text{ g protein}/1 \text{ g N}} - \left[\left. \frac{\text{(Urinary urea}}{\text{nitrogen}} \right/ 24 \text{ hr} + 3.5 \right) \right]$$

Example: NB = $\frac{56 \text{ g protein}}{6.25}$ − (8.0 g urea N + 3.5)

= 8.96 g N − (8.0 g urea N + 3.5)

= 8.96 g − (11.5 g N)

= −2.54 g N

= Negative nitrogen balance

FIG. 9. Formula for calculating nitrogen (N) balance. (Adapted from refs. 5 and 24.)

used in the formula in Fig. 9 is based upon information from Blackburn (4,5) and the "Recommended Dietary Allowances" (23).

Creatinine Height Index

The creatinine height index is an indicator of lean body mass or muscle tissue (3,4,5,7,9,15,25,30). Creatinine is excreted at a constant rate in the urine regardless of the diet (3,9,15,30), but the amount of creatinine excreted depends upon the amount of lean body mass a person has (3,30). If a patient is malnourished he has probably lost lean body mass, as well as adipose tissue. As a result his creatinine excretion is lowered and the creatinine height index is decreased (9).

It is necessary to obtain a 24-hr urine collection sample to calculate the creatinine height index. This urine sample must be as accurate as possible (9,15), because the validity of the creatinine height index depends upon this factor (15). Special attention must also be paid to kidney function tests and to treatments that alter kidney function (9), since a disturbance in the glomerular filtration rate alters the amount of creatinine excreted in the urine (9).

The creatinine height index (Fig. 10) is a comparison of the

$$\text{CHI } (\%) = \frac{\text{mg creatinine/24 hr} \times 100 \text{ excreted by patient}}{\text{mg creatinine/24 hr excreted by person of same height at ideal weight}}$$

Example:
$$\text{CHI} = \frac{675 \text{ mg (patient)} \times 100}{1{,}035 \text{ mg (ideal)}}$$
$$= 0.652 \times 100$$
$$= 65\% \text{ of standard}$$

FIG. 10. Creatinine/height index (CHI) of lean body mass. Female 5′6″. (Adapted from refs. 5 and 30.)

TABLE 3. *Ideal urinary creatinine values*[a]

Adult men[b]		Adult women[c]	
Height (cm)	Ideal creatinine (mg)[d]	Height (cm)	Ideal creatinine (mg)[d]
157.5	1,288	147.3	830
160.0	1,325	149.9	851
162.6	1,359	152.4	875
165.1	1,386	154.9	900
167.6	1,426	157.5	925
170.2	1,467	160.0	949
172.7	1,513	162.6	977
175.3	1,555	165.1	1,006
177.8	1,596	167.6	1,044
180.3	1,642	170.2	1,076
182.9	1,691	172.7	1,109
185.4	1,739	175.3	1,141
188.0	1,785	177.8	1,174
190.5	1,831	180.3	1,206
193.0	1,891	182.9	1,240

[a] Adapted from ref. 3.
[b] Creatinine coefficient (men) = 23 mg/kg ideal body weight.
[c] Creatinine coefficient (female) = 18 mg/kg ideal body weight.
[d] Total 24 hr.

amount of creatinine excreted in 24 hr by the patient with the estimated excretion of creatinine by a person of the same height at ideal body weight (3,30). Tables (Table 3) have been developed that give the ideal creatinine excretion values for adult men and adult women at ideal body weight for various heights (3).

Delayed Hypersensitivity Skin Testing

Delayed hypersensitivity skin testing is used in evaluating the cellular immune response (2,4,19,27). It has been found that the immune response of a protein-calorie malnourished person is depressed and can be improved with proper nutrition (2,19).

Delayed hypersensitivity skin testing involves injecting an antigen subcutaneously into the forearm (Fig. 11) (27). Several antigens are available for skin testing (4,27). The induration, and sometimes erythema, at each injection site are measured at

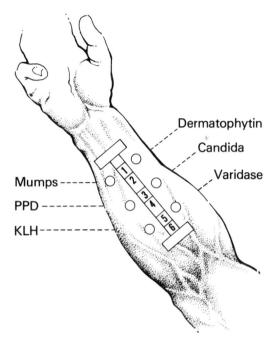

FIG. 11. Delayed hypersensitivity skin testing.

24 and 48 hr (27). Usually, the greater the induration, the more intact the immune system (4,27). Classifications for grading the intensity of response vary among researchers (4,27). It is important to research the literature and consult the immunologists at a specific institution to determine response classifications for that patient population.

The delayed hypersensitivity reaction of cancer patients is being evaluated as a prognostic indicator (13,28). It is hoped that, in the future, the effect of adequate nutrition upon delayed hypersensitivity response will be investigated. This will help in determining the impact adequate nutrition has upon maintenance of immune status in cancer patients.

CONCLUSIONS

Making a nutritional assessment of the cancer patient is a challenge because of the complexities of the disease and the complexities in its treatments. The tools currently used for nutritional assessment provide a practical method for assessing nutritional status; however, at present there is no reliable method for establishing the nutritional needs of the cancer patient (11).

Cancer patients are among the most rewarding patients for the dietitian to work with. The cancer patient can benefit from nutritional counseling and assistance from the day of his diagnosis, and over the many months and years he may be receiving treatment. It is important to remember that the purpose of nutritional assessment is to assist the dietitian and physician in developing an individualized nutritional care plan, and to provide the objective follow-up information necessary in adjusting the nutritional care plan to meet the patient's changing needs.

REFERENCES

1. Balogh, M., Kahn, H., and Medalie, J. H. (1971): Random repeat 24-hour recalls. *Am. J. Clin. Nutr.*, 24:304–310.
2. Bistrian, B. R., Blackburn, G. L., Scrimshaw, N. S., and Flatt, J. B. (1975): Cellular immunity in semistarved states in hospitalized adults. *Am. J. Clin. Nutr.*, 28:1148–1155.
3. Bistrian, B. R., Blackburn, G. L., Sherman, M., and Scrimshaw, N. S. (1975): Therapeutic index of nutritional depletion in hospitalized patients. *Surg. Gynecol. Obstet.*, 141:512–516.
4. Blackburn, G. L., and Bistrian, B. R. (1976): Nutritional support resources in hospital practice. In: *Nutritional Support of Medical Practice*, edited by H. A. Schneider, C. E. Anderson, and D. B. Coursin, pp. 139–151. Harper and Row, New York.
5. Blackburn, G. L., Bistrian, B. R., Maini, B. S., Schlamm, H. T., and Smith, M. F. (1977): Nutritional and metabolic assessment of the hospitalized patient. *J. Parenteral and Enteral Nutr.*, 1:11–22.
6. Blackburn, G. L., Maini, B. S., Bistrian, B. R., and McDermott, W. (1977): The effect of cancer on nitrogen, electrolyte, and mineral metabolism. *Cancer Res.*, 37:2348–2353.
7. Butterworth, C. C., and Blackburn, G. L. (1975): Hospital malnutrition. *Nutrition Today*, March–April:8–18.
8. Christakis, G., editor. (1974): *Nutritional Assessment in Health Programs*. American Public Health Association, Washington, D.C.
9. Committee on Procedures for Appraisal of Protein-Calorie Mal-

nutrition of the International Union of Nutritional Sciences (1970): Assessment of protein nutritional status. *Am. J. Clin. Nutr.,* 23:807–819.

10. Costa, G. (1977): Cachexia, the metabolic component of neoplastic disease. *Cancer Res.,* 37:2327–2335.
11. Costa, G. (1977): Determination of nutritional needs. *Cancer Res.,* 37:2419–2424.
12. Davidsohn, I., and Henry, J. B., editors (1974): *Todd-Sanford Clinical Diagnosis by Laboratory Methods,* pp. 653–656. W. B. Saunders, Philadelphia.
13. Eilber, F. R., and Morton, D. L. (1970): Impaired immunologic reactivity and recurrence following cancer surgery. *Cancer,* 25: 362–367.
14. Forbes, G. B. (1973): Another source of error in the metabolic balance method. *Nutr. Rev.,* 31:297–300.
15. Forbes, G. B., and Bruining, G. J. (1976): Urinary creatinine excretion and lean body mass. *Am. J. Clin. Nutr.,* 29:1359–1366.
16. Frisancho, A. R. (1974): Triceps skin fold and upper arm muscle size norms for assessment of nutritional status. *Am. J. Clin. Nutr.,* 27:1052–1058.
17. Jelliffe, D. B. (1966): *The Assessment of the Nutritional Status of the Community.* World Health Organization, Geneva.
18. Kremer, W. B., and Laszlo, J. (1973): Hematologic complications of cancer. In: *Cancer Medicine,* edited by J. F. Holland and E. Frei, III, pp. 1085–1099. Lea and Febiger, Philadelphia.
19. Law, D. K., Dudrick, S. J., and Abdou, N. I. (1973): Immunocompetence of patients with protein-calorie malnutrition: The effect of nutrition repletion. *Ann. Intern. Med.,* 79:545–550.
20. Lindner, P., and Lindner, D. (1973): *How to Assess Degrees of Fatness.* Cambridge Scientific Industries, Cambridge, Maryland.
21. Mackenzie, T. A., Blackburn, G. L., and Flatt, J. P. (1974): Clinical assessment of nutritional status using nitrogen balance. *Fed. Proc.,* 23:683.
22. Madden, J. P., Goodman, S. J., and Guthrie, H. A. (1976): Validity of the 24-hour recall. *J. Am. Diet. Assoc.,* 68:143–147.
23. National Academy of Science. (1974): *Recommended Dietary Allowances,* 8th edition, Washington, D.C.
24. Ohnuma, T., and Holland, J. F. (1977): Nutritional consequences of cancer chemotherapy and immunotherapy. *Cancer Res.,* 37: 2395–2406.
25. Sauberlich, H., Dowdy, R. P., and Skala, J. H. (1974): *Laboratory Tests for the Assessment of Nutritional Status,* pp. 93–98. CRC Press, Cleveland.
26. Seltzer, C. C., and Mayer, J. (1977): Greater reliability of the triceps skin fold over subscapular skin fold as an index of obesity. *Am. J. Clin. Nutr.,* 20:950–953.

27. Sokal, J. E. (1975): Measurement of delayed skin test responses. *N. Engl. J. Med.,* 293:501–502.
28. Sokal, J. E., and Aungst, C. W. (1971): Cellular immune responses and prognosis in the malignant lymphomas. *Natl. Cancer Inst. Monogr.,* 34:109–112.
29. Validity of 24-hour dietary recalls, (unsigned) (1976): *Nutr. Rev.,* 34:310–311.
30. Viteri, F. E., and Alvarado, J. (1970): The creatinine height index: Its use in the estimation of the degree of protein depletion and repletion in protein-calorie malnourished children. *Pediatrics,* 46:696–706.
31. Young, V. R. (1977): Energy metabolism and requirements in the cancer patient. *Cancer Res.,* 37:2336–2347.

Nutritional Management of the Cancer Patient, edited by J. Wollard.
Raven Press, New York © 1979.

Nutritional Management with Radiotherapy

Carolyn Thornton

Department of Nutrition and Food Service, The University of Texas System Cancer Center M. D. Anderson Hospital and Tumor Institute, Houston, Texas 77030

Nutritional problems associated with radiation therapy depend on (a) the part of the body involved in the treatment field (see Table 1); (b) the intensity of tumor dose received; (c) the time over which a radiation dose is administered; (d) the volume of tissue irradiated; and (e) the patient's nutritional status at the beginning of treatment. For radiation to be optimally effective, and for healing of normal tissues to occur, the patient must consume enough calories and protein to maintain body weight despite uncomfortable reactions and adverse side-effects. This is not something that the average patient will automatically do, but requires much education and encouragement from the dietitian, physician, nurse, social worker, family members, and all others involved in the patient's care.

Patients most often tending to develop nutritional problems are those presenting with cancers of the oral cavity, including tongue, floor of mouth, upper and lower gingivae, hard palate, and buccal mucosa, and those who have tumors involving the larynx, nasopharynx, or hypopharynx. Neck nodes are frequently present under these conditions. Patients with this type of cancer mainly are heavy smokers and/or heavy drinkers, although this is not always the case. There may be a history of malnutrition due to typical poor eating habits, and vitamin B and C deficiencies secondary to smoking and drinking. In addition, the tumor itself may discourage eating due to pain upon

43

TABLE 1. *Nutritional problems according to part of body irradiated*

Head and neck
1. Dry mouth
2. Loss or change in taste
3. Difficulty swallowing
4. Loss of appetite
5. Sore mouth and throat

Esophagus
1. Difficulty swallowing
2. Sore throat
3. Fistulas
4. Obstruction

Lung
1. Loss of appetite
2. Shortness of breath
3. Sore throat
4. Nausea

Upper abdomen
1. Nausea
2. Vomiting

Whole abdomen
1. Nausea and vomiting
2. Cramping and gas
3. Diarrhea

Pelvis
1. Diarrhea

attempting to eat, or difficulty in swallowing. If the patient has undergone surgery for tumor removal, he may have incurred weight loss due to physical impairment from the surgery itself. Indeed, it is an exceptional patient who presents at the start of radiation therapy in excellent nutritional health.

The major problems encountered by the patient undergoing radiation to the head and neck area, however, are due to the adverse reactions to irradiation. Normal tissues in the treatment field are affected as well as neoplastic cells. Reactions that occur and affect eating and nutrition include:

1. Dry mouth, due to involvement of major salivary glands

in the treatment field. Mucous becomes scant and thick, making swallowing difficult, and foods may feel as though they are "sticking" in the throat. For some patients, this feeling also produces nausea. This effect may occur as early as three or four days after treatment begins (see Fig. 1).

2. Change in or loss of taste, probably due to "radiation-induced damage to the microvilli of the taste cells, or to their surfaces" (1). A study conducted by Conger (1) demonstrated that loss of taste is "exponential and rapid." After 3 to 3½ weeks of radiation, patients in the study could barely detect as sweet a sugar solution as the equivalent to about 25 teaspoons sugar/teacup, as acid a solution as 50% household vinegar, or as bitter a quinine solution as one concentrated 1,500 times more than bottled "quinine water." Loss of taste comes as a bewildering problem to many patients. Food is described as tasting "rancid" (particularly red meats), like "wood," "cardboard," or "cotton." It is understandable that appetites begin to wane. If patients try to force foods down regardless, often they will experience nausea.

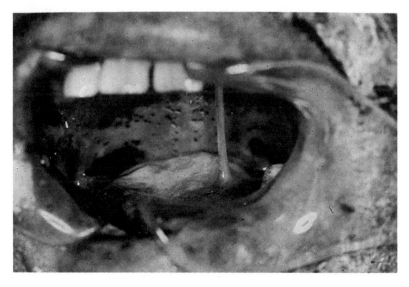

FIG. 1. Dry mouth.

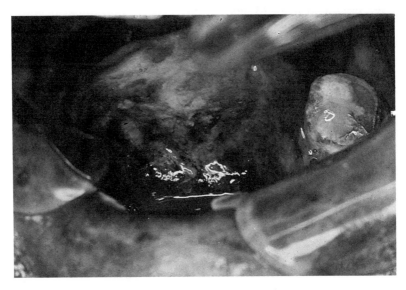

FIG. 2. Mucositis and ulcerations.

3. Sore mouth and throat. Sometime in the second or third week of treatment, patients begin to experience pain and a burning sensation in the mouth and/or throat. This is due to radiation reactions including erythema, mucositis, or ulcerations (Fig. 2). Occasionally infections are present to further complicate the picture. Pain is intensified when the patient attempts to eat. Swallowing becomes especially difficult, particularly if edema is also present. It is at this point that the unmotivated patient will decrease his intake of food and beverages, or else his diet becomes limited to perhaps two or three items. Weight loss, negative nitrogen balance, and further damage to normal mucosa will occur rapidly without nutritional intervention.

NUTRITIONAL MANAGEMENT OF PATIENTS WHO HAVE TUMORS OF THE HEAD AND NECK

The usual tumor dose for patients who have tumors of the head and neck is 5,000 to 6,000 rads given over a period of 5 to 6 weeks. It is important for the dietitian to get to know the patient and his family as soon as possible after treatment begins. A number of factors are to be considered (Table 2). Since the majority of patients are treated on an outpatient basis, it becomes necessary to learn whether the patient is a resident of the city or is staying at a hotel, motel, rented apartment, rehabilitation center, or with friends or relatives. This will make a difference as to how much a patient can do for himself, i.e., whether or not he will be able to fix between-meal high protein beverages, or will have to depend upon canned nutritional supplements. Occasionally a patient will have no kitchen or refrigeration facilities, and will have to eat all meals in a cafeteria or restaurant. Whether the patient is alone or with supportive friends or relatives is worthy of consideration. The encouragement of a loving wife, husband, daughter, or other significant person when the going gets rough, can make a great deal of difference as to whether or not a patient is able to maintain his weight and nutritional status.

Recent changes in the patient's weight, dietary habits, or appetite are important information for the dietitian. For example, is the patient anorexic? Does he have a history of weight loss or gain? Food allergies and preferences play an important role, also. Can the patient tolerate milk? Does he like eggs? Is he on a special diet of any kind? The initial interview with the patient should reveal answers to all these questions and more. Individualization is extremely important.

For instruction of patients who have tumors of the head and

TABLE 2. *Considerations made when dealing with nutritional problems*

1. Patient's living condition
2. Patients food habits, likes, and dislikes
3. Food allergies, aversions, or intolerances
4. Recent weight changes and contributing factors
5. Support from others
6. Previous nutritional knowledge

neck, a list of simple behavioral objectives has been set up. The patient is expected to:

1. Understand why nutrition is important during treatment.
2. Be able to recognize high protein food sources.
3. Be able to recognize high calorie food sources.
4. Be familiar with possible adverse reactions from radiation therapy, and how to cope with them.

The patient is first given a list of ordinary foods such as roast beef, honey, macaroni, chicken, cottage cheese, buttermilk, yogurt, rice, spinach, etc. The patient is asked to mark those foods he likes and eats, and then to indicate which foods are high in protein. This is a simple exercise, but from it the dietitian can get an idea of how much the patient already knows about nutrition and thus gear the instruction accordingly. A brief diet history can give the dietitian more information on the patient's nutrition knowledge, food habits, allergies, likes and dislikes, etc. It is very important for the interviewer to ask lots of questions at this point and to listen to the answers very carefully.

At the M. D. Anderson Hospital, each patient with head and neck cancer receives a copy of the booklet entitled "Nutrition for Cancer Patients Receiving Radiation Therapy" (4). This booklet contains basic nutrition information, plus a sample meal plan, and recipes for high-calorie, high-protein beverages. Anticipated reactions are also described, along with a number of helpful suggestions for dealing with each problem.

After going through the booklet, patients can use the food list again to test for and to reinforce knowledge gained. For example, the patient can then mark foods that would add calories to his diet. He can state how he is going to modify his current eating habits when swallowing becomes difficult. Positive reinforcement for each correct statement is used liberally. An encouraging, positive attitude on the part of the instructor is very helpful and seems to be contagious. A patient who says, "I'm going to do all I can to keep my weight up," usually will!

The initial instruction is, of course, only the beginning. Patients are seen on a regular basis until the end of treatment. They are weighed daily and many take pride in gaining a few pounds initially. As problems occur, specific dietary modifications are suggested. These include changes in texture, consistency, portion sizes, etc., as necessary. Many times the job is simply listening to the patient and lending encouragement and support. Repetition is necessary and beneficial. Some frequent specific suggestions are as follows:

For dry mouth: Patients are encouraged to increase fluid intake, attempting to drink a total of at least 2 quarts of fluid/day. Water is good, since its composition is similar to saliva, but a higher-calorie beverage may also be necessary. Patients are advised to keep water or other beverages on hand for sipping when needed. Foods are more easily swallowed when moistened with sauces, gravies, or broth. Small sips of liquids taken with bites at meals also make swallowing easier. Patients are also told to avoid breathing through the mouth. Chewing sugar-free gum or sucking on sugar-free hard candy may also help to stimulate salivation. (Saliva is a natural protection against cavities. With its decrease, teeth are more susceptible to damage, thus, retentive sweets are not encouraged.) An artificial saliva swished through the mouth several times per day is also beneficial in relieving the discomfort of dry mouth.

For change in taste: Patients are encouraged to experiment with different flavors and seasonings. For example, some patients report being able to taste lemon flavored foods for longer periods. The person who does the cooking is asked to make certain the meal is attractive, and ways of achieving this goal are discussed. Many times if foods look appealing, the patient is able to eat regardless of whether he can actually taste the food. Some patients benefit from trying to remember what the food ordinarily tastes like. As for taste aversions, patients are advised to avoid those foods which tend to nauseate them. Red meats tend to taste "spoiled" before chicken or fish. Later in treatment, cheese or egg products may be largely substituted for meats for better acceptance. Many patients report aversions to sweet foods. They may dilute sweet liquids with milk to make them taste bland. Some patients drink bland tube-feeding formulas mixed with various flavorings such as instant coffee. Occasionally, a patient will add a pinch of salt to a too-sweet drink, as this is found to be just enough to cut down the sweetness and provide an acceptable product.

For loss of appetite: Patients are asked to eat small meals, but more of them. Six to eight small meals per day are often easier to consume and digest than larger meals. Patients are encouraged to keep high-calorie, high-protein snacks on hand for between-meal snacking. An eggnog product is provided by the M. D. Anderson Radiotherapy Department for patients to drink while waiting for treatment. Quart containers are also available so that the product may be carried home. Even those patients who have no kitchen or refrigeration facilities can keep the eggnog product on hand in a small ice chest. Samples of canned nutritional supplements are also kept on hand for the patients to try. These products are available for purchase at the hospital pharmacy or in selected drugstores in the area.

For sore mouth and throat: Patients are instructed to eat soft, nonacidic foods. If swallowing becomes extremely difficult, foods may need to be blended or liquefied. The American Cancer Society provides two blenders to be kept on hand in our department, which may be loaned to patients during their treatment period. Recipes for blended foods and high-protein, high-calorie beverages are available. Patients are advised that foods are more comfortable to irritated mouth and throat tissues if eaten at room temperature rather than very hot or very cold. The use of a straw may also prove beneficial in taking liquids.

The patient requires much encouragement during these difficult periods. Of benefit to him are oral irrigations of a salt-soda solution (1 teaspoon salt and 1 teaspoon soda to 1 quart lukewarm water), which can be given before and after each meal or snack and upon arising in the morning. Local anesthetics such as lidocaine are also available. Some patients find relief by chewing aspirin-containing gum. Systemic pain killers may also be prescribed, if necessary.

If, in spite of all efforts, the patient is simply not able to eat enough to maintain hydration and nourishment, a tube may be inserted and tube feeding begun to insure proper healing. Patients may elect to use a commercial tube-feeding formula or may prefer to make their own formula at home. Recipes providing adequate amounts of nutrients are given for home-made formulas.

A few patients have been hospitalized and fed parenterally due to severe reactions to treatment or physical impediments contraindicating tube feeding. However, nutrition via the enteral route is still much preferred.

It is important not to overlook discharge planning for these patients. They need to be aware that the mouth and throat will remain sore for approximately 2 weeks after treatment, and that a high-calorie, high-protein intake is still very important for maximum healing to take place. Complete return of taste takes much longer, anywhere from 2 to 4 months (1), although some patients report that it never totally returns. Dryness of the mouth can also be a persistent problem. An encouraging, supportive attitude on the part of the dietitian and others involved in discharge planning is important.

NUTRITIONAL MANAGEMENT WITH RADIOTHERAPY TO OTHER PARTS OF THE BODY

Many of the same interviewing and instructional techniques are used in dealing with nutritional problems occurring due to radiation therapy to other parts of the body. However, to avoid repetition, they will not be outlined in detail. Generally, a "balanced" diet containing adequate amounts of protein is recommended, with modifications in composition, texture, consistency, etc., made as necessary. Weight maintenance is stressed for all patients undergoing radiotherapy, even for those occasional patients who are overweight.

Esophagus

Patients with tumors of the esophagus often experience severe weight loss due to difficulties in swallowing. Individual differences are present, but most patients are able to consume very soft or blended foods. Occasionally a patient will be able to ingest only liquids. In any of these situations, patients need instruction on preparation of foods or beverages, frequency of feedings, and nutritional content of food products consumed. Once again, radiation treatment will produce damage to the mucosa, possibly resulting in esophagitis or even fistula. A gastrostomy, or jejunostomy tube feeding may need to be initiated to assure the ingestion of adequate calories and protein. Hyperalimentation has also proven helpful in management of patients with obstructing carcinomas of the esophagus (2).

Lung

It is quite common to observe patients with lung cancer who have had up to a 20-pound weight loss over a short period of time. Loss of appetite and shortness of breath are seen as contributing factors. The dietitian should initiate a nutritional build-up program early in the course of treatment. Radiation to this area may produce some throat soreness and difficulty in swallowing. Occasionally nausea is also a problem. Patients are instructed on high-calorie, high-protein, soft, blended or liquid diets with emphasis on between-meal supplements. Treatment plans vary, but many bronchogenic patients receive 10 to 15 treatments, are then allowed a rest period of 3 to 4 weeks, and then given 10 to 15 more treatments. Many patients experience burning and soreness in the throat and esophagus during their rest period. Patients need to be made aware that this reaction is common, and suggestions for dealing with it are given.

Upper Abdomen

Abdominal radiation is frequently given to patients with lymphomas. The most common side effect from treatment to this area of the body is nausea and vomiting. Patients differ as to how severely they are affected. Specific dietary tips on management of nausea and vomiting are given (covered in more detail in another chapter) along with much encouragement. Antiemetic drugs such as chlorpromazine are also useful. As always, weight maintenance is stressed.

Whole Abdomen

On occasion, the whole abdomen, including the pelvis, may be irradiated. The whole area can be treated at the same time, or a "moving strip" method may be employed (Fig. 3). With

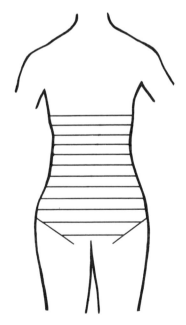

FIG. 3. "Moving strip" technique.

this method, "strips" 2.5 cm apart are marked off on the patient's body, front and back. The "strips" can be treated individually, moving down the patient's body, until eventually the whole area is treated. This method of treatment is commonly used with ovarian cancers, some lymphomas, and seminomas involving the abdominal cavity (3). Nutritional problems are frequent when the radiation field covers the whole abdomen, due to such a large area of the gastrointestinal tract involved. Nausea and vomiting may be present, but there is also the possibility of diarrhea. For patients receiving the "strip" type of radiation, diarrhea generally occurs when the pelvis is treated, and nausea when the upper abdomen is treated. With radiation to the whole abdomen, the intestinal mucosa may be damaged with resulting flattening of the villa, thus decreasing the area available for absorption of nutrients. There is also a decrease in enzymes, many of which are normally located on the surface of the villa. Patients who are undergoing whole abdominal or strip-technique radiation are given instruction early in the course of treatment on a restricted-residue, high-protein diet. A high-protein intake is important to aid in stabilization of blood counts (6). Small, frequent meals are encouraged, with emphasis on fluid, potassium, and sodium intake. A list of low-residue snack foods is given to each patient. Such items as smooth peanut butter on crackers, hard-boiled eggs, mild cheddar cheese, marshmallows, juices and nectars are encouraged between meals for calories to remain high enough to maintain body weight. A restricted lactose diet may also be indicated since lactose can be destroyed by radiation. Medications such as diphenoxylate-atropine are used to help control diarrhea. Low lactose, low residue supplemental products may be sampled and used on a regular basis if they prove helpful. Some patients may benefit from the use of an elemental diet. A low-fat diet may also be helpful, as malabsorption of fat in abdominal radiation has been described in some studies (5).

With all these restrictions, it has still been possible for patients to maintain weight and consume adequate nutrients if carefully monitored. A multivitamin supplement is advised as insurance against possible deficiencies.

Pelvis

If the radiation field covers the pelvis alone, many of the above considerations apply, due to the possibility of diarrhea. Cancers of the cervix, bladder, or prostate are frequently involved. Severity of the problem will depend on the volume of tissue irradiated and the length of the treatment. If the treatment lasts longer than 3 weeks, diarrhea may generally be expected. In this case, a restricted-residue, high-protein diet is advised, with caution given in regard to lactose and fat intake.

Colon and Rectum

Colorectal cancer patients are given instruction on a restricted-residue, high-protein diet early in the course of their treatment. It is especially important that diarrhea be controlled in this group, as irritation to the colostomy stoma is a very painful and aggravating complication.

In summary, nutrition is a very important consideration for patients receiving radiation therapy. Fortunately, at M. D. Anderson Hospital the physicians and other staff in the Department of Radiotherapy are well attuned to this fact and lend much support to the patient as well as reinforcement to dietary measures employed by the dietitian. Much effort and cooperation is provided by all involved in the patient's care in order to keep nutritional problems to a minimum, so that the treatment modality of radiation may provide its maximum benefit to the cancer patient.

REFERENCES

1. Conger, A. D. (1973): Loss and recovery of taste acuity in patients irradiated to the oral cavity. *Radiat. Res.,* 53:338–347.

2. Copeland, E. M., and Dudrick, S. J. (1976): Intravenous hyper-alimentation as adjunctive treatment in the cancer patient. *Clinical Digest,* Vol. 5, Number 1.

3. Delclos, L., and Smith, J. P. (1975): Ovarian cancer, with special regard to types of radiotherapy. *National Cancer Institute Monograph,* 42:129–135.

4. Heaton, C. A. (1977): Nutrition for cancer patients receiving radiation therapy. M. D. Anderson Hospital publication, Houston, Texas.

5. Sobo, A. O., and Johnston, I. (1973): The effect of therapeutic irradiation of the abdomen on intestinal absorption of man. *Am. J. Gastroenterol.,* 60:616–624.

6. St. John Elliott, C. (1976): Radiation therapy: How you can help. *Nursing '76,* 6:34–41.

Nutritional Management of the Cancer Patient, edited by J. Wollard.
Raven Press, New York © 1979.

Nutritional Consequences of Cancer Surgery in Patients Who Have Neoplastic Diseases

Debra A. Buchanan

Department of Nutrition and Food Service, The University of Texas System Cancer Center M. D. Anderson Hospital and Tumor Institute, Houston, Texas 77030

The physiological stress of surgery places added nutritional demands upon the well-nourished patient. The presurgical patient with cancer who often presents with anorexia, poor nutritional intake, and an undesirable weight is thus at an even greater risk to have a complicated postoperative course. A discussion of the patient's presurgical and postsurgical nutritional demands will assist in defining the role of the clinical dietitian in the nutritional assessment and management of the patient undergoing surgery for cancer.

Optimum nutritional status is a worthy goal in any presurgical patient. The body's reactions to stress, the healing of wounds, and infection control depend upon the homeostasis of body fluids and tissue (8). The increase in the rate of wound infection and the increased hazard of pulmonary complications in the obese surgery patient is proven. Conversely, in the malnourished, underweight patient, host resistance to infection may be impaired by starvation and vitamin and protein deficiencies (1). Therefore, the nutritional status of the patient should be assessed preoperatively using his weight, biochemical profile, and dietary profile as parameters. The patient's nutritional care plan may include weight gain or reduction. Because many patients who have neoplasms need to gain weight or increase biochemical values, such as low serum albumin, before surgery, the following discussion will be devoted to nutritional build-up.

The type of nutritional build-up to be used (enteral versus parenteral) must be determined by the clinical situation. There are advantages and disadvantages to both. If nutritional build-up needs to be rapid or if the patient cannot take food by mouth due to anorexia, stomatitis, or obstruction, or cannot have tube feeding due to low platelets, intravenous hyperalimentation (IVH) is often considered. However, enteral hyperalimentation has its advantages. Rowlands et al. (7) suggest that the nitrogen-sparing effect of protein and calories is greater when given via the gastrointestinal tract rather than intravenously, as greater amounts of protein and calories are needed proportionately to achieve nitrogen balance by the i.v. route. Prolonged intravenous hyperalimentation may significantly decrease the patient's appetite; this becomes particularly important when trying to convert the patient back to taking food by mouth. However, patients receiving enteral hyperalimentation require careful biochemical monitoring just as do those on IVH to prevent glycosuria, osmotic diuresis, and dehydration (4).

The following modes of enteral nutritional build-up are available:

1. Regular food by mouth plus supplement (i.e., Sustacal in addition to regular foods or Polycose added to foods)
2. Complete nutritional supplement (i.e., Ensure or Nutri-1000)
3. Tube feeding (i.e., homemade pureed, Isocal, Compleat B)
4. Tube feeding plus supplement (i.e., Isocal with Polycose)
5. Elemental diet (i.e., Flexical or Vivonex) either by tube or by mouth

Postsurgically, these same modes of enteral hyperalimentation may be used to ensure a desirable nutritional status despite increased metabolic demands. Researchers have indicated that about 0.1 g of nitrogen and 20 kCal/kg/day are needed to restore body tissue during early convalescence (6). The apparent inactivity associated with convalescence is often deceptive; even though the patient appears to be at rest, his body is responding catabolically and anabolically to the initial stress. As a result, his caloric requirements can be increased 50% or more.

The catabolic phase is characterized by a decreased appetite and decreased peristalsis with an increase in temperature and pulse rate. When the turning point is achieved, appetite usually is regained; peristalsis is stimulated and normalization of temperature, pulse, and biochemical values occurs. An adequate supply of carbohydrate, fat, protein, vitamins, minerals, and fluid is necessary for this phase and the subsequent anabolic phase to take place. After needed protein is resynthesized in the anabolic phase, the body gradually regains lost fat (2). Wound healing and possible infection and fever are factors also contributing to the rise of energy requirements. With fever, there is an estimated 7.2% increase in caloric expenditure for every degree Fahrenheit increase in body temperature (12).

Only a small portion of the debilitated patient's nutritional requirements is satisfied through the use of routine isotonic parenteral feeding regimens. One liter of 5% dextrose solution, which contains 50 g carbohydrate, will provide only 200 kCal. Thus, with the limits of fluid overload taken into consideration, a patient who receives 3,000 ml of 5% dextrose in water a day will obtain only 600 kCal. It then becomes apparent that adequate alimentation needs to be initiated as soon as possible. The sometimes established pathway of prolonged parenteral fluids, clear-liquid diet, etc., may not be adequate for the increased nutritional demands of the surgical patient. If the patient must be kept on liquids for an extended period, then a high-calorie, high-protein liquid diet with nutritional supplementation of commercial products such as Sustacal or Ensure, is indicated (2). Commercial or homemade nutritional preparations can also be used when the patient is on solid food, as between-meal feedings, to further increase caloric intake.

Many postsurgical patients may be scheduled to take chemotherapy or radiation therapy, or both, and their nutritional status will be stressed even more in the future. The type of nutritional support rendered depends upon the type of cancer surgery performed and its subsequent nutritional consequences. A discussion of these potential nutritional consequences will further emphasize the need for preoperative and postoperative nutrition intervention. Refer to Table 1 for a summary of these postsurgical nutritional problems.

The head and neck presurgical patient often presents with weight loss and poor nutritional intake, due to impaired mastication and alcoholism. Enteral nutrition in the form of oral nutrition supplementation or tube feeding and/or IVH may achieve weight gain or a desirable increase in presurgical biochemical values. Surgery involving the alimentary canal makes nasogastric tube feedings initially necessary after surgery in order that healing may take place in the affected area. The sub-

TABLE 1. *Nutritional consequences of "radical" resection*[a]

Organs resected	Nutritional sequellae
Oral cavity and pharynx	Dependency on tube feedings
Thoracic esophagus	Gastric stasis (secondary to vagotomy) Fat malabsorption Gastrostomy feedings in patients without reconstruction
Stomach	Dumping syndrome Fat absorption Anemia
Small intestine	
Duodenum	Pancreatobiliary deficiency with fat malabsorption
Jejunum	Decrease in efficiency of absorption (general)
Ileum	Vitamin B_{12} and bile salt malabsorption
Massive (> 75%)	Fat malabsorption and diarrhea; vitamin B_{12} malabsorption; gastric hypersecretion
Colon (total or subtotal)	Water and electrolyte loss

[a] From ref. 5, with permission.

ject of tube feedings (types, initiation, tolerance, etc.) will be discussed in another chapter. Gradually, the head and neck patient may be advanced to liquids, pureed foods, soft foods, and so on, by mouth. Often nutrition rehabilitation may be involved as the patient learns to chew and swallow with partial or no tongue, mandible, palate, or teeth and learns to change long-standing poor dietary habits. The dietitian as well as other members of the health-care team are a source of encouragement and assistance in this area. No matter what consistency diet the patient is able to tolerate, the dietitian should be sure he is ingesting a variety of nutrients in sufficient quantities to maintain weight and biochemical values.

Esophagectomy often may induce significant malabsorption of fat since removal of vagus nerves results in steatorrhea and gastric atony. The fecal fat losses that occur can be compensated for by an increase in caloric intake, frequent small meals, and the exchange of medium chain triglycerides for long chain fatty acids in the diet (5,10). When the esophagus is not reconstructed, patients may depend upon gastrostomy tube feeding as a source of nutrition.

Nutritional problems may be more frequently encountered after partial or total gastrectomy for cancer than after esophagectomy. This impairment includes some metabolic defects due to malabsorption, as well as various symptom problems that may limit total intake. The normal stomach serves as a reservoir to receive and retain food, alter the food to some degree by digestive processes, and slowly discharge the altered food into the small intestine at a rate that is most efficient for the digestive and absorptive functions of the gut. Thus, major mechanical changes in the size of the stomach, or its emptying function, may have a great impact on nutritional capabilities of the patient. The nutritional problems observed after gastric resection generally increase proportionately with the extent of the resection. The primary defect in absorption that may play a role in chronic difficulties with weight maintenance and nutrition in the postgastrectomy patient is impairment of fat absorption. However, all of the measurable fecal fat losses after gastrectomy can be balanced by increasing fat intake, as the percentage of fat absorbed remains constant over a wide range of intake. Associated problems in absorption of iron, vitamin B_{12}, and calcium also may occur, but deficiencies of these may be prevented by oral supplementation or, in the case of vitamin B_{12}, injections.

Postprandial symptoms after radical gastrectomy play a major role in malnutrition by producing a self-limited intake of food-stuff related to what is termed the "dumping syndrome." The symptoms of the "dumping syndrome" include epigastric fullness, hyperperistalsis, cramps, nausea, vomiting, and/or diarrhea. High carbohydrate meals, which are more likely to become hyperosmolar, intensify symptoms of dumping in patients who have had gastrectomies. A high-protein, high-fat, low-carbohydrate, frequent-feeding dietary regimen has been shown to be beneficial in reducing the possibilities of dumping syndrome. This diet eliminates a high carbohydrate insult to the small bowel while reducing the sudden influx of food in large quantities into the bowel by using small, frequent feedings. The increased fat component of the diet provides adequate calories in as small a volume as possible. Not only is there higher caloric value of fat/gram, but both protein and fat have the additional advantage of slower enzymatic breakdown in the bowel than carbohydrate, thereby avoiding the rapid development of a hyperosmolar solution in the bowel (5). Patients should have their intervals between meals and content of their postgastrectomy diet individually assessed. The time needed for adherence to a special diet depends upon the tolerance and progress of each patient.

Emphasis on optimal nutrition in patients who have bowel resections cannot be overlooked. Malabsorption of certain nutrients will depend on amount and area resected. The ability of various segments of the small intestine to increase their absorptive capabilities prevents major clinical problems after small bowel resection, except for those patients who have had massive bowel resections (in the range of 75% of the total small bowel).

The fecal fat losses can be much greater after bowel resection than after gastrectomy. Persistent gastric secretion can lead to acid diarrhea, and electrolyte and water imbalance. In those patients who do require resection of more than 2 feet of ileum and the ileocecal valve, there may be a significant increase in fecal fat, but this may be controlled with a high-protein, low-fat diet. Vitamin B_{12} injections are required to correct a vitamin deficiency that results from resection of this bowel segment. Resection of up to 8 feet of the jejunum fails to interfere with the absorption of glucose, fat, protein, folic acid, vitamin B_{12} or other vitamins, but resection of both the jejunum and ileum is accompanied by an increase in absorptive problems with all nutrients. The diarrhea and increased fecal calcium, magnesium, and other electrolyte losses occurring in some patients with massive resection may be reduced by exchanging long-chain fatty acids for medium-chain triglycerides in the diet. Elemental diets begun at low concentrations are tolerated well via a small feeding tube by the anorexic patient. This alternative meets nutritional requirements until the patient can tolerate food by mouth. Thus, the dietitian, keeping in mind the type of bowel resection that patients have had and the possible nutritional problems they might encounter (Fig. 1), can suggest appropriate alimentation, feeding methods, and nutrient supplementation. Please refer to the chapter on ostomies for a comprehensive discussion of the nutritional care of the colostomy patient.

The pancreatectomy patient also poses numerous nutritional problems. Preoperative weight loss is a very common presentation. For this reason, nutrition build-up prior to surgery is stressed. As with this and other surgeries, nutrition build-up can often be carried out enterally up until the day before surgery if low-residue elemental liquid nutrition is used. Pancreatectomy due to carcinoma leads to diabetes and malabsorption of amino acids, calcium, magnesium, fat-soluble vitamins, and vitamin B_{12}. With more severe surgery requiring partial removal of the stomach along with the pancreas, more complications are likely. Diabetic diets along with the use of pancreatic enzymes and

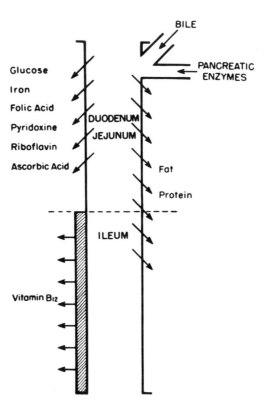

FIG. 1. Sites of normal absorption from the small intestine. (From ref. 5, with permission.)

small amounts of insulin are required to help control the problem. Good control of the diabetes enhances carbohydrate utilization and minimizes fluid and sodium losses secondary to osmotic diuresis caused by glycosuria. Medium-chain triglycerides are usually better absorbed by the pancreatectomy patient (11).

Ureterosigmoidostomy is the implantation of the ureters into the sigmoid colon following removal of a malignant bladder. Because of the metabolic problems of this procedure, it has been replaced with the ureteroileostomy or ileal conduit. An ileal conduit is a way of diverting urine outside the body when the urinary bladder has been removed. A short section of the small intestine is resected to form a conduit with no change in bowel movements. The patient is fitted with an appliance that collects urine outside the body. Since treatment of bladder cancer often involves presurgical pelvic irradiation, patients may experience bowel damage, poor food intake, and weight loss. This, combined with the stress of surgery, may place the patient in poor nutritional status unless nutritional considerations are made (11). Often a high-calorie, high-protein elemental diet given orally or by tube may be used before surgery to improve nutritional status. Other nutritional supplements used after surgery will aid in weight maintenance. Weight maintenance is important with any ostomy patient in order that his appliance may fit and function well.

Achieving ideal weight prior to surgery may be of particular concern to the dietitian who is working with overweight or underweight gynecology and breast patients. Postoperative patients may need continued nutrition counseling regarding ideal weight maintenance. Gynecology patients who have bowel resections and/or ostomies may have some of the nutritional problems, including weight loss, mentioned previously. Frequently, postsurgical gynecology patients receiving chemotherapy or radiation therapy will need nutritional counseling regarding a restricted-residue, restricted-fat, multiple feeding regimen using low residue nutritional supplements such as Vivonex or Precision LR. This regimen appears to reduce diarrhea and malabsorption, thus contributing to weight stabilization or gain.

Breast cancer patients may have several important postsurgical nutritional considerations. Patients with advanced disease and metastases may manifest hypercalcemia. Because there is a controversy over whether dietary calcium significantly contributes to serum calcium, a restricted-calcium diet may or may not be implemented. Schneider and Sherwood (9) suggest that, in the great majority of cases where hypercalcemia derives mainly from the skeleton, dietary restrictions have limited effects. It should be pointed out that calcium-containing foods such as milk are a very important source of calories for many underweight patients. To restrict this nutrient might be compromising the patient's weight for little or no effectiveness in controlling blood calcium.

A recent study by Donegan, et al. (3) suggests that excessive body weight may contribute to the recurrence of breast cancer after surgical treatment. Thus, weight reduction by dietary means may improve the prognosis of overweight individuals with early stages of breast cancer.

In conclusion, the dietitian working with cancer surgery patients has four major objectives:

1. To strive for ideal weight maintenance and desirable biochemical and dietary profiles before and after surgery, keeping in mind the type of surgery performed and its potential nutrition consequences.

2. To try to make the patient's diet as nutritionally complete as possible by utilizing those foods he can tolerate, together with nutritional supplements and/or vitamin and mineral preparations. If food by mouth cannot be tolerated, tube feeding or IVH are alternatives.

3. To communicate with physicians, nurses, and other staff regarding the patient's nutritional needs.

4. To continue to follow patients and offer encouragement and reinforcement for their proposed nutritional care plans.

REFERENCES

1. Altemeier, W. A. (1976): *Manual on Control of Infection in Surgical Patients,* p. 68. American College of Surgeons, J. B. Lippincott Co.
2. Bresner, M. (1977): Nutrition for the surgical patient. *J. Oral Surg.,* 35:200–203.
3. Donegan, W. L., Hartz, A. J., and Rimm, A. A. (1978): The association of body weight with recurrent cancer of the breast. *Cancer,* 41:1590–1594.
4. Kaminski, M. V., Jr. (1976): Enteral hyperalimentation. *Surg., Gynecol., Obstet.,* 143:12–16.
5. Lawrence, W., Jr. (1977): Nutritional consequences of surgical resection of the gastrointestinal tract for cancer. *Cancer Res.,* 37:2379–2385.

6. Moore, F. D. (1971): Convalescence: The metabolic sequence after injury. In: *Manual of Preoperative and Postoperative Care*, edited by J. N. Kinney, R. H. Egdahl, and G. D. Zuidema, p. 19. W. B. Saunders, Co., Philadelphia.
7. Rowlands, B. J., et al. (1977): Nitrogen sparing effect of different feeding regimens in patients after operation. *Br. J. Anaesth.*, 49: 781–787.
8. Sabiston, D. C., Jr., editor. (1972): *Textbook of Surgery*, p. 116. W. B. Saunders, Co., Philadelphia.
9. Schneider, A. B., and Sherwood, L. M. (1974): Calcium homeostasis and the pathogenesis and management of hypercalcemia disorders. *Metabolism*, 23(10):975–1007.
10. Shils, M. E. (1976): Nutritional problems in cancer patients. In: *Nutrition in Disease*, pp. 13–16. Ross Laboratories, Columbus, Ohio.
11. Shils, M. E. (1977): Effects on nutrition of surgery of the liver, pancreas, and genitourinary tract. *Cancer Res.*, 37:2387–2394.
12. Stahl, W. M. (1972): *Supportive Care of the Surgical Patient*, p. 42. Grune and Stratton, Inc., New York.

Nutritional Management of the Cancer Patient, edited by J. Wollard.
Raven Press, New York © 1979.

Chemotherapy and Nutritional Management

Nancy L. Fong

Department of Nutrition and Food Service, The University of Texas System Cancer Center M. D. Anderson Hospital and Tumor Institute, Houston, Texas 77030

Therapeutic approaches to cancer treatment produce a variety of side effects that directly affect the patient's nutritional status. The potential nutritional complications, along with the biochemical and histological trauma of major organ systems, may leave the patient with profound nutritional insufficiencies (10). To prevent nutritional deficiency and to treat nutritional consequences, the dietitian must manage the patient's symptomatic complications, maintain his optimal nutritional health, and provide continual supportive therapy.

Chemotherapy, surgery, irradiation therapy, and immunotherapy are the major modalities utilized in the treatment of cancer. During the past quarter decade, chemotherapy has assumed a major role in the early treatment of the disease. Recent advances in new drug development, and combination chemotherapy and adjuvant chemotherapy with surgery and irradiation, have contributed to chemotherapy's increased use.

Since cancer is a disease of the cells, the battle between cancer and chemotherapy takes place within the cell structure. The goal of chemotherapy is to control the growth of, or destroy completely, cancer cells by interfering with cell doubling and destroying the malignant cells (2). All the cancer cells must be destroyed to achieve a cure. This goal has not been reached to date with most malignancies; however, a high rate of tumor regression with an improved rate of survival may be achieved, accompanied by lessened symptoms and improved patient well-being.

Chemotherapy acts at the cellular level to directly kill tumor cells (cytocidal action) or to induce adverse conditions that prevent tumor cell replication (cytostatic action) (7). Cell cycle models have been developed to demonstrate this action. An abbreviated model (see Fig. 1) shows four phases: G_1, S, G_2, and M. G_1, the first growth period, is the phase in which enzymes, structural proteins, and cell organelles are synthesized. During the S phase, DNA synthesis takes place. G_2 is the second growth period. In the M phase, cell division, or mitosis takes place (15). In planning chemotherapy schedules the principle consideration is that of timing. Chemotherapy is most effective during cell division when the cell is most sensitive to cytotoxic drugs. However, precise timing is difficult, since a consistent cycling time for a specific cell population has not been determined (1).

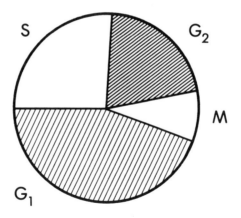

S = DNA Synthesis
M = Mitosis (Division)
G_1 = First Growth Period
G_2 = Second Growth Period

FIG. 1. Cell cycle model.

The various antineoplastic agents affect different stages of the cell life cycle (1). Some affect the cell during one or more phases, but have no adverse effects on the cell during the other phases. These are called "cell-cycle specific" drugs. Cell-cycle specific drugs work best during proliferation phases of the cell cycle. Copeland and Dudrick have speculated that if one used intravenous nutritional support to stimulate multiplication of cancer cells during these phases, the cell-cycle specific drugs might totally eliminate the cancer from the host (4).

Resting tumor cells are not affected by cell-cycle specific agents but are sensitive primarily to alkylating agents and antibiotics, which also attack the cells in other phases of the cycle (7). These drugs, called "cell-cycle nonspecific," have prolonged action regardless of the phase of cell cycle. Each chemotherapy dose kills some of the neoplastic cell population.

Skipper documents the need for cells to be well nourished for the antineoplastic agent to achieve maximum effect (14). DNA synthesis can be halted, for example, during conditions when uracil is lacking, or essential amino acids unavailable (14). Both healthy and malignant cells need protein synthesis for mitosis to occur (8). The response to all cancer treatment, and especially chemotherapy, has been shown to be greater when a patient is in a good nutritional and biochemical status, whereas cachetic patients have lower therapeutic safe margins for most cancer treatments (3).

CLASSIFICATION AND ADMINISTRATION OF DRUGS

Antineoplastic drugs are classified according to their structure and their biochemical mechanism. A common classification includes five basic categories:

1. Alkylating agents
2. Antimetabolites
3. Natural products

A. *Vinca* alkaloids
B. Antibiotics
4. Miscellaneous
5. Hormones
A. Adrenocorticosteroids
B. Sex hormones

Depending on the drug, chemotherapeutic agents are administered by four major routes: intramuscularly, subcutaneously, orally, and intravenously. The patient's tolerance of the drug and his body surface area are used to determine the dosage of each drug. Body surface area is calculated from his height and weight measurements, and chemotherapy doses are computed on a milligram per m^2 basis, to assure a dose proportionate to the patient's size. When drugs are used in combination, the dosage for each drug is lower than when it is used alone.

Several goals in drug selection for combination treatment include:

1. Selecting drugs that are effective when used alone.
2. Combining drugs that work together instead of inhibiting each other's action in the cell cycle.
3. Utilizing drugs with different mechanisms of action in the cell cycle.
4. Combining drugs that produce a different toxicity at different times.

The choice of agent and administration plan are dependent on the type of cancer and the protocol used. Criteria for selecting patients, requirements for monitoring patients, and general directives to the investigators are included in protocols used by clinicians.

Chemotherapy is not a continuous process, since cancer is a chronic disease that is not treated in a single visit to the clinic or hospital. Often, patients undergo several days of drug therapy as outlined in a course of treatment. A drug-free interval is usually scheduled between courses, to allow time for repair of normal tissue, time for complete resolution of side effects, and valuable time for nutritional buildup.

MANAGING SIDE EFFECTS

What the health care team knows about chemotherapy determines how well the team can help the patient adjust to the circumstances of treatment. A patient seems to cope with the side effects of therapy better if he understands the treatment

TABLE 1. *Common side effects of chemotherapy*

System involved	Side effect
Gastrointestinal	Nausea
	Vomiting
	Diarrhea
	Constipation
	Dyspepsia
	Heartburn
	Ulceration
	Mucositis
Muscle and nerve	Weakness
	Lethargy
	Tingling, numbness
Bone marrow	Anemia
	Infection secondary to decreased white cells
	Thrombocytopenia
Skin and mucosal	Dermatitis
	Stomatitis
	Skin pigmentation
	Alopecia, partial or complete
Urinary tract	Hemorrhagic cystitis
	Colored urine
	Decreased renal function
Reproduction	Amenorrhea
	Impaired spermatogenesis
Miscellaneous	Fever, chills
	Malaise
	Poor appetite, weight loss

plan. The patient should, therefore, take an active role in his own treatment, helping the clinician detect toxic reactions. The patient should understand in advance the meaning of individual tolerance and possible reactions to each drug or treatment.

Symptoms or side effect are frequently seen with commonly used chemotherapy drugs. Their effects can take a toll on the well-being of each patient, as shown in Table 1.

Until recently, weight loss was accepted as an unavoidable consequence of chemotherapy. This is no longer the case, because techniques and systems have been discovered that control the symptoms that lead to weight loss.

NAUSEA AND VOMITING

Nausea and vomiting are the problems most frequently associated with chemotherapy. Some of the nausea is psychological

TABLE 2. *Tips on the dietary management of nausea and vomiting associated with chemotherapy*[a]

1. Carbonated beverages such as Coke, Sprite, or ginger ale can help curb nausea.

2. Use small frequent meals to prevent prolonged empty stomach.

3. After periods of sleep or rest, dry crackers or toast, eaten before activity begins, help curb nausea.

4. Tart foods such as lemons and dill or sour pickles may also help control nausea.

5. Popsicles and gelatin desserts increase fluid intake and are satisfying.

6. Smell sensitivities are often altered during chemotherapy. Cold meat plates, sandwiches, fruit plates, cottage cheese, and other cold foods offer good nutrition without having an overpowering aroma which often cause nausea.

7. Medications can easily alter taste sensations, making foods that are normally favorites taste differently. Select foods that are appealing and, if the taste is not as expected or is undesirable, try another food.

8. Relax and chew foods well to prevent and/or minimize anxiety and a tense stomach.

[a] Some chemotherapy drugs may produce side effects of nausea and vomiting. The presence and severity of these side effects will vary with the individual patient. The above are general guidelines that have been helpful to many patients at M. D. Anderson Hospital in counteracting these side effects.

in origin, but is physically real to the patient. Nausea and vomiting are common with patients receiving antibiotics, alkylating, or antimetabolite agents. Antiemetics are used liberally, frequently in conjunction with mealtimes, but the antiemetics presently available are not always totally effective in controlling drug-induced vomiting (10). See Table 2 for tips in the management of nausea and vomiting.

DIARRHEA

Diarrhea commonly affects the patient receiving antibiotics and antimetabolites. Prolonged uncontrolled diarrhea results in dehydration, electrolyte imbalance, and accelerated malnutrition (10). To combat diarrhea, small frequent meals low in roughage are encouraged. Rich, spicy, and gas-forming foods should be avoided. Patients should increase fluid intake and eat foods rich in potassium.

CONSTIPATION

Constipation is a sign of neuropathy and must be controlled before further complications occur. Often constipation may result from eating a softer or more liquid diet than the patient is accustomed to. Roughage or fiber should be increased in the diet, and food should be chewed thoroughly. If the diet must be soft, bran added to cooked cereals and casseroles and grated raw fruits and vegetables may be helpful.

STOMATITIS

Another side effect the cancer patient may encounter is stomatitis (Fig. 2), resulting from antimetabolite and antibiotic drugs. Stomatitis, which may be an early sign of toxicity, is an inflammation of the muscous membrane and may affect the tongue, palate, gums, and floor of the mouth. The rapid turnover of epithelial cells may be the reason for such sensitivity

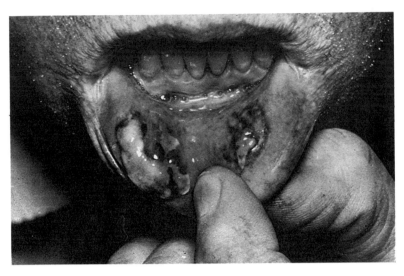

FIG. 2. Stomatitis.

10,12). Patients with these inflamed ulcerations have a varying degree of food tolerance.

Generally cold, soft, nonacidic foods are best tolerated. Tilting the head back or using a straw may make swallowing more comfortable. If the pain is severe, the physician may recommend a topical anesthesia such as lidocaine (Xylocaine®) or warm saline mouth irrigations every 4 to 6 hr (11). The patient should be cautioned to be aware of extreme temperatures of foods when a topical anesthesia is used, since a patient may receive burns without realizing it.

ANOREXIA

Anorexia, a side effect of many cancer states, is one of the most difficult symptoms to treat. Anorexia may be caused by psychological, emotional, or treatment-induced factors and complications, but often the cause is the disease itself as it progresses (17). Depression, especially at the time of initial diagnosis or when the disease recurs, may further decrease a desire for food. The patient may also develop conditioned responses if he suffers from nausea and abdominal pain after eating (5).

A number of hypotheses have been offered regarding possible causes of anorexia. Although no direct supporting evidence has been presented as yet, Theologides has suggested that the hypothalamus may be involved. He posits that neoplasms may produce a humoral factor that acts upon the hypothalamus' regulatory centers for hunger and satiety (16). The effect is compounded by a decreased taste acuity (hypogeusia), perverted sense of taste (dysgeusia), and decreased smell acuity (hyposmia) induced by chemotherapy. Another hypothesis suggests that chronic use of certain antineoplastic drugs causes hepatotoxicity, inducing anorexia (18). With hepatic anorexia, the anorexia progresses during the day, which is why breakfast is usually the best meal of the day for these patients (18).

Regardless of its cause, a vicious cycle of disease–therapy-related malnutrition can be detrimental to the patient (9). Treatment of anorexia and improvement of the patient's metabolic condition may contribute to the patient's sense of well-being, improve his response to therapy, and diminish the toxicity of treatment.

Patients with anorexia and early satiety should be encouraged to eat small, frequent, highly nutritious meals at a leisurely pace. Relatives should be instructed to only "encourage," not "force," patients to eat. Mealtimes should be made enjoyable, using pleasant odors and textures and favorite foods to stimulate the patient's appetite. The patient's cravings for certain foods should be satisfied if possible. High-protein, high-calorie supplements should be available. Modification of eating is based on principles of behavior modification, and is discussed in another chapter.

ALTERED TASTE PERCEPTION

Changes in taste perception are noted with many cancer patients, particularly an elevated threshold for sweet and a lowered threshold for bitter tastes (6). Cancer patients need a higher-than-normal level for sweet before they detect it. Once the detection level has been reached, however, the patient population at M. D. Anderson Hospital has generally found that additional sweetness quickly becomes intolerable. Many nutritional supplements must therefore be altered by using additions, such as instant coffee or fruit juices, to mask the sweetness. The lower threshold for bitterness may be the reason why many patients develop an aversion to meat. Patients having difficulty consuming meats usually have the most problems tolerating beef and pork but may be able to tolerate fish and poultry. Patients are encouraged to incorporate into their diets other protein foods such as dried beans, eggs, and cheese as substitutes for meat.

Altered taste perception can be managed with the use of extra seasonings and spices, as tolerated. Acid foods stimulate the taste buds and are recommended as a part of each meal. As with anorexia, appealing textures, an attractive setting, and colorful foods are helpful in making meals more appealing. It has been suggested that patients who respond to cancer therapy tend to find their taste sensitivities return to normal (11).

NUTRITION EDUCATION

Patients often can develop nutritional deficiencies and malnutrition, not from the side effects of treatment, but rather by following a dietary regimen in which they avoid so called "carcinogenic" foods or by consuming large amounts of foods alleged to be "healthful." Nutrition information, and sometimes misinformation is abundantly available in many popular magazines and books. It is important to combat misinformation and to guide the patient in proper nutritional care, using such resources as video tapes, organized classes, and pamphlets. These instructional aids can help the patient, his family members, and his friends understand the side effects of treatment, and can teach them management techniques.

NUTRITION ASSESSMENT

The effects of cancer on host tissue and whole-body energy metabolism are only partially understood, so it is impossible to recommend precisely the minimum intake of energy and nutrients sufficient to meet the energy need and maintain body energy balance in cancer patients (19). However, normal cellular function is important for successful cancer treatment (4).

Caring for a cancer patient on chemotherapy can challenge a dietitian's nutritional skills. She must be able to establish a data

TABLE 3. *Basic nutritional care plan*

I. Assessment
   A. Height
   B. Weight
      1. Body weight change in relation to time
      2. Consideration of possible edema or ascites
   C. Change in bowel habits
   D. Dietary history
      1. Food habits
      2. Altered food preference; food aversions
      3. Meal patterns
      4. Nutrient intake
   E. Review of biochemical profile
      1. Serum albumin
      2. Hemoglobin
      3. Hematocrit
      4. Blood sugar
      5. Iron
      6. Electrolytes
      7. Skin test response
   F. Evaluation of absorption ability

II. Planning with health care team

III. Implementation
   A. Initiate nutritional support
   B. Monitor response

IV. Evaluation
   A. Note improvement or change in assessment factors
   B. Note patient response
   C. Alter plan if desired response is not met

base, assess the patient, and follow the most effective plan of action (Table 3).

Nutritional goals during chemotherapy include:

1. Achieve minimal weight loss.
2. Correct or forestall nutritional imbalances and/or deficiencies (17).

Daily weights of the patient receiving chemotherapy should be recorded for signs of dehydration or weight loss. It is ironic that during therapy, when a patient needs to be in the best possible nutritional state, he may well be at his worst, because of the therapy's side effects. Often commercially prepared nutritional supplements are suggested at this time. This topic is discussed in detail in another chapter.

With complications of nausea, vomiting, and diarrhea, the patient's fluid and electrolyte balance must be carefully monitored and replenished. If a patient is taking Cytoxan or Isophosphamide, fluid is even more important. These drugs can cause hemorrhagic cystitis if the patient does not take in and retain enough fluids. During chemotherapy, the constituents of cells, including purines, are released into the blood stream. These purines are converted into uric acid, elevating blood urea nitrogen. To speed excretion of uric acid and decrease the hazard of crystal and urate stone formation, the patient must increase fluid intake (2). Three liters of fluid a day are recommended. Since many cancer patients have difficulty maintaining weight, high caloric beverages to replenish fluids are suggested. Carbonated beverages, popsicles, juices, etc., add both fluid and nutrients.

AFTER CHEMOTHERAPY

The nutritional goals following chemotherapy include increased appetite and weight gain, if any has been lost during the course of drug treatment. Usually the patient's appetite will improve spontaneously following completion of treatment. He will tolerate small high protein, high-calorie meals with between-meal supplements better than he will the standard three meals a day.

A balanced diet incorporating a variety of foods should be encouraged at this time. If lack of variety for mechanical, physical, or psychological reasons is a problem, a therapeutic multi-vitamin supplement is suggested to insure adequate intake of all nutrients.

Chemotherapy is becoming a commonplace, standard practice in the treatment of cancer. Today the trend is towards early drug treatment to prevent the spread of disease in patients with minimal cancer. Along with early diagnosis, early treatment, and new diagnostic and therapeutic regimens, nutritional support is recognized as important in greater patient response and, therefore, in improved survival rates (3,13). To help the patient reach and maintain optimal health, it is essential to be familiar with practical means of managing his nutritional requirements during and after chemotherapy.

REFERENCES

1. Bingham, C. A. (1978): The cell-cycle and cancer chemotherapy. *Am. J. Nurs.*, 78:201–205.
2. Burns, N. (1978): Cancer chemotherapy a systemic approach. *Nursing '78*, 8:57–63.
3. Copeland, E. M., Daly, J. M., and Dudrick, S. J. (1977): Nutrition as an adjunct to cancer treatment in the adult. *Cancer Res.*, 37:2451–2456.
4. Copeland, E. M., and Dudrick, S. J. (1975): Cancer: Nutritional concepts. *Semin. Oncol.*, 2:329–335.
5. DeWys, W. D., and Herbst, S. H. (1977): Oral feeding in the nutritional management of the cancer patient. *Cancer Res.*, 37:2429–2431.
6. DeWys, W. D., and Walter, K. (1975): Abnormalities of taste sensation in cancer patient. *Cancer*, 31:1888–1896.
7. Golden, S. (1975): Cancer chemotherapy and management of patient problems. *Nurs. Forum*, 16:278–289.
8. Hoffman, J., and Post, J. (1973): The effects of antitumor drugs on the cell cycle. In: *Drugs and the Cell Cycle*, edited by A. M.

Zimmerman, G. M. Padilla, and I. L. Cameron, pp. 219–247. Academic Press, New York.

9. Krumdieck, C. L. (1974): Nutrition and Cancer. *Ala. J. Med. Sci.,* 11:153–154.

10. Ohnuma, T., and Holland, J. (1977): Nutritional consequences of cancer chemotherapy and immunotherapy. *Cancer Res.,* 37:2395–2405.

11. Schein, P. S., MacDonald, J. S., Waters, C., and Haidak, D. (1975): Nutritional complications of cancer and its treatment. *Sem. Oncol.,* 2:337–347.

12. Shils, M. E. (1972): Nutritional problems arising from the treatment of cancer. In: *Nutrition and Cancer.* American Cancer Society, New York.

13. Shils, M. E. (1977): Enteral nutrition by tube. *Cancer Res.,* 37:2432–2439.

14. Skipper, H. E. (1971): Cancer chemotherapy is many things. *Cancer Res.,* 31:1173–1180.

15. Taylor, N. B., editor (1973): *Best and Taylor's Physiological Basis of Medical Practice,* ninth edition, pp. 4–13. Williams and Wilkins Company, Baltimore.

16. Theologides, A. (1974): The anorexia-cachexia syndrome: A new hypothesis. *Ann. N.Y. Acad. Sci.,* 230:14–22.

17. Theologides, A. (1976): Anorexia-producing intermediary metabolites. *Am. J. Clin. Nutr.,* 29:552–558.

18. Theologides, A. (1977): Nutritional management of the patient with advanced cancer. *Postgrad. Med.,* 61:97–101.

19. Young, V. R. (1977): Energy metabolism and requirements in the cancer patient. *Cancer Res.,* 37:2336–2347.

Nutritional Management of the Cancer Patient, edited by J. Wollard.
Raven Press, New York © 1979.

Anorexia in the Cancer Patient

Janice Johnson

Department of Nutrition and Food Service, The University of Texas System Cancer Center M. D. Anderson Hospital and Tumor Institute, Houston, Texas 77030

The anorexia of malignancy occurs when the nutritional requirements of the host and tumor are not satisfied by food intake. Since a patient's voluntary food consumption can be limited by factors other than cancer, such as nausea and other disorders related to eating, it is important to distinguish between a patient's absence of hunger and his distaste for food (5).

Anorexia and cachexia occur commonly in man and laboratory animals with cancer (2,4,16). Anorexia is often one of the first symptoms of neoplasia; the resulting weight loss may be one of the first indications that the patient should consult a physician (4,14). Anorexia is also one of the first causes of cachexia in a patient with a tumor (11). Cancer cachexia is primarily the result of abnormality in the regulation of food intake (5,10). Cachexia is one of the leading causes of death in cancer patients (16).

Studying the anorexia and cachexia of cancer patients presents several problems. Since the physical deterioration that occurs in the cancer patient is not caused exclusively by a reduction in food intake, there is no simple correlation between anorexia and cachexia (4,16). Variables in tumor, patient, and treatment may, therefore, interfere with the study of anorexia. Tumor variables include the location, size, and growth rate of the tumor and the areas of metastasis. Relevant patient variables are nutritional status before the onset of the disease and the

83

results of decreased food intake. In treatment, variables may affect assimilation and metabolism of the food (7).

The effect of a tumor upon loss of appetite is most evident prior to diagnosis, before therapeutic and psychological factors become significant (17). Anorexia is not related in any way to the size or type of cancer (4), but does increase in frequency and severity in more advanced stages of the disease (18).

The observation that appetite and weight loss in cancer patients have frequently been due to causes other than intestinal obstruction, endocrine abnormalities, or the presence of pathogenic organisms, has led to the belief that the tumor can produce alterations in the patient's metabolism (13). The effects of starvation, for example, appear to be greater upon a tumor-bearing host than on a non-tumor-bearing host (2). Although information is lacking concerning the specific effects of a tumor upon metabolism (8), we do know that the disease or its treatment produces an increase in energy expenditure (3,14). Researchers have proposed several explanations for this increased energy expenditure. One suggestion is that the continuous growth of malignant tissue requires more energy than the growth of normal tissue (14). Another explanation is that the tumor may initiate nutritional deficiencies, producing deviations in intermediary metabolic functions of the patient and resulting in the use of pathways that demand more energy and nutrients (5,14). The use of certain metabolites by the tumor may also cause some biochemical reactions to be unavailable to the patient (14). The presence of a tumor may cause abnormalities in the patient's oxidative and energy-conserving systems (14).

A reduction in food intake, lassitude, apathy, and a further decline in food intake is a familiar cycle in cancer patients (2). The resulting poor nutritional status interferes with a patient's response to various forms of treatment, such as surgery, chemotherapy, and radiotherapy (12,18). A number of factors contribute to patient anorexia, e.g., the regulation of hunger and satiety, the taste of food, and the patient's psychological reaction to the disease and its treatment.

REGULATION OF HUNGER AND SATIETY

Normally, food consumption is regulated by the body's satisfying metabolic requirements with food intake, if food is available. Alterations in food intake can occur as a result either of a change in feeding activity, measured by duration, or of feeding efficiency, measured by quantity of food ingested per unit of feeding activity. Rats with transplanted tumors reduce the duration of meals and, later, the frequency. Morrison (10–12) has observed that the feeding efficiency of rats with tumors increases to compensate for a decline in feeding activity so that food intake remains constant. As the disease progresses, however, feeding efficiency and meal frequency decrease along with feeding activity, resulting in a reduction in food intake.

A similar pattern exists in human cancer patients, who reach satiety quickly, even when they were hungry before eating (16). This is why small, frequent feedings, rather than three large meals per day, can be more easily tolerated by the anorectic patient (18).

The pathogenesis of anorexia is not fully understood. One might assume that anorexia could be explained by disorders in the mechanisms that regulate hunger and satiety (17). However, not enough information is available concerning these mechanisms, so that some aspects of the physiology of hunger and satiety are still hypothetical (15). Several theories have been proposed to explain the regulation of food intake. Since food intake may not be significantly influenced by a single disorder, DeWys (7) has suggested that anorectic patients may have several abnormalities in their hunger and satiety regulatory systems. Areas where abnormalities could occur are discussed below.

Hypothalamus

The hypothalamus is the primary center of the brain for regulating food intake, with ventromedial nuclei being "satiety" centers and lateral nuclei being "feeding" centers (5,7,15). Its role in regulating appetite and satiety has been illustrated by experiments involving the bilateral destruction of both the lateral and ventromedial hypothalamus. Anorexia and starvation result from lesions in lateral hypothalamic nuclei, whereas the destruction of ventromedial nuclei induces polyphagia and obesity (17).

The relationship between anorexia in cancer patients and the hypothalamic centers is not fully understood. Both tumor-induced anorexia and reduced food intake have been recognized in a significant number of cancer patients, leading to research on the hypothalamic regulation of food intake (2). After recovery from lesions of the lateral hypothalamus, animals become more selective in their food, avoiding foods that had earlier been acceptable (5). DeWys (7) has suggested that the stress of the disease may stimulate the release of substances that suppress feeding behavior.

Destruction of the lateral or ventromedial hypothalamus has not been convincingly shown to modify cachectic development in laboratory animals. Therefore tumor growth may have a greater effect on factors that are stimulated extra-hypothalamically than on those that are stimulated hypothalamically (10,12), indicating a less-than-clear relationship between anorexia and the hypothalamus.

Alimentary Tract

The oropharyngeal region, neuroreceptors in the stomach, and baroreceptors and chemoreceptors in the intestine regulate food intake by sending signals for satiety after consumption of a particular amount of food (15). It has been suggested that a tumor may interfere with appetite by releasing toxic polypeptides that depress gastrointestinal mucosal cells. However, lack of experimental evidence for this hypothesis suggests that sensations from the alimentary tract do not perform a primary function in the regulation of food intake (15,17).

Thermostatic Regulation

It has been postulated that the "specific dynamic action" of food, or the heat liberated during its absorption, performs a regulatory function in food intake (7,15). The additional energy expenditures of individuals with tumors result in additional energy requirements (14).

The release of heat from the oxidative phosphorylation of liver mitochondria could account for the anorexia of cancer. However, there is no indication that alterations occur either in energy-producing reactions or in the coupling mechanisms of individuals with tumors (15).

A cold environment causes a temporary increase in food consumption in anorectic tumor-bearing rats, indicating their significant need to satisfy the requirements for heat production in spite of the anorectic effects of a malignancy (7,15).

Glycostatic Regulation

The theory of glycostatic regulation is based on the supposition that blood glucose functions as a link between the supply of nutrients and the hypothalamus. It has been suggested that hypothalamic glucoreceptors are stimulated by the rate of glucose utilization, not by blood glucose values (7,15).

Cancer patients have exhibited abnormalities of carbohydrate metabolism similar to those of subclinical diabetes patients, as indicated by a decreased rate of glucose utilization (5,7,15). Since satiety depends on the rate of glucose utilization, however, one might anticipate the increase in appetite that is evident in diabetes, rather than anorexia (15,17).

Lipids

Body lipids with sensors for free fatty acids and glycerol perform a regulatory function in food intake (7). Hypothalamic centers control the stability of body fat stores and may be linked to total body fat by a steroid (15). Since neoplastic cells can produce steroids, the suggestion has been made that the tumor uses these steroids to satisfy its metabolic needs, but that they may interfere with appetite (5).

Osmoreceptors

Dehydration of tissue caused by the transport of water from intracellular to extracellular compartments produces signals of satiety (15,17). Since the tissues of cancer patients have a high content of water, however (4,14), an increased, rather than a decreased appetite would be expected if predictions were based on water content of tissues (15).

Hormones

Insulin, growth hormone, glucagon, enterogastrone, and cholecystokinin have been identified as having functions in the regulation of food intake (7,15). Clinical observations indicate that increased appetite and food intake are stimulated by administration of adrenal corticosteroids (15) or increased serum insulin (7,10). Since the production of adrenal corticosteroids is increased in cancer, an increased appetite might be predicted (15). However, a simultaneous decline in insulin production observed in cancer patients could be a cause of suppressed appetite (7).

Amino Acids

Food consumption is considered to be regulated in part by the concentration and pattern of amino acids in the blood and extracellular fluids (7,15). Elevated levels of amino acid nitrogen, protein split products, and amino acids have been found in the blood of tumor-bearing animals and of humans with cancer (5,15). Cancer patients also exhibit abnormalities in urinary excretion of amino acids (14). The anorexia of cancer may, therefore, be partially accounted for by alterations in amino acid patterns (7,15).

Nutrient Deficiency

It had been suggested that the anorexia of cancer results from the absence of a certain nutrient sufficient to satisfy the requirements of both tumor and patient (5,15). Two observations would seem to refute this. First, no excessive amounts of a nutrient have been found in malignant neoplasms. Second, except for the utilization of glucose by malignant masses, excessive consumption of any particular nutrient has not been identified in metabolic studies (15).

Pituitary Peptides

The observation of anorectic peptides in the urine of patients with advanced malignancies has resulted in the assumption that anorexia may be produced by cancer-caused polypeptides, oligonucleotides, and other low molecular weight metabolites (5,7,15). The peptides and other small metabolites may produce anorexia by causing the satiety and feeding centers in the hypothalamus and other parts of the central nervous system to depress appetite and stimulate satiety (17).

TASTE

The taste of food has a significant effect upon its palatability, particularly when such other factors as nausea and the psychological aspects of cancer interfere with food acceptance. There is a relationship between changes in taste sensation and suppressed food intake (7).

Cancer patients are often dissatisfied with the taste of food. DeWys (6) has observed a general reduction in the pleasurable aspect of taste among patients with malignancies. Cancer seems to produce unsatisfactory changes in taste thresholds (18). The most significant change appears to be the lower threshold for bitter-tasting foods, which is probably responsible for the aversion to the taste of meat and other high-protein foods frequently observed in cancer patients (2,6,12,18).

The thresholds commonly used in taste experiments are the thresholds of detection and recognition. The detection threshold is the lowest concentration at which a patient can taste a solution as being different from water, while the recognition threshold involves the patient's ability to identify the solution as tasting sweet, bitter, sour, or salty (3). The sweet, bitter, sour, and salty thresholds are tested using sucrose, urea, dilute hydrochloric acid, and sodium chloride, respectively (3,6,12).

Experiments involving taste thresholds in cancer patients should select subjects very carefully, since abnormalities in taste can be due to many variables unrelated to the disease. Among the factors affecting taste acuity are smoking, other diseases, medications, highly modified diets, and alcoholism (3).

Carson and Gormican (3) observed that before cancer patients are treated with the chemotherapeutic agent 5-fluorouracil, their taste abnormalities included a decreased sensitivity to salt and sweet tastes, but no change in bitter or sour thresholds. Experiments conducted after chemotherapy indicate a variety of changes in patients' taste acuity, possibly determined by sex, type of cancer, and extent of the disease. After treatment, changes in taste acuity are greater among men than women, among colon cancer patients than breast cancer patients, and among those in whom the disease is more advanced (3).

It has been suggested that elevated taste thresholds might be due to a reduction in the number of taste bud cells. A possible explanation for a lower taste threshold for bitter foods might be the subthreshold stimulation of taste buds by abnormal blood levels of amino acids (6).

Radiation to the oropharyngeal area can destroy a patient's sense of taste, resulting in "mouth blindness" and affecting food acceptance (8,13). A dry mouth, produced by the anticholinergic effect of some chemotherapeutic agents also reduces taste (12). Because tastelessness results in anorexia, the appearance and smell of food become more important to the cancer patient (13).

The return to normal taste thresholds seems to depend upon a patient's response to antineoplastic therapy. Taste acuity tends to return to normal if therapy causes a reduction in tumor size (6,12).

The need for additional research in the area of taste has been suggested by DeWys (6) and Morrison (12). Such studies of taste acuity, indicating that taste abnormalities require dietary modifications, have resulted in recommendations designed to improve food acceptance in cancer patients (3,18).

PSYCHOLOGICAL CAUSES AND EFFECTS

Holland et al. (9) divide the anorexia of cancer into three categories. Anorexia can be related to emotional distress, to therapeutic procedures, or to various stages of the disease itself. In order to determine the appropriate nutritional management of anorexia, it is important to identify the psychological factors that may influence its occurrence or its severity at any given stage of the disease.

Anorexia Caused by Emotional Stress

Emotional distress is a typical reaction to circumstances involving a life-threatening illness. Anorexia is one of several symptoms that may indicate the effect of emotional stress upon a person undergoing diagnostic tests for cancer. The knowledge that he has cancer may disrupt a patient's normal daily pattern of activities. Therefore, any weight loss occurring at this time may be psychologically induced and not attributable to the cancer itself (9).

Once the diagnosis of cancer has been made, emotional and psychological responses of the patient may either produce anorexia or intensify it (3,17), supporting the suggestion that the central nervous system can reduce appetite in response to psychological reactions to illness (5).

Anorexia can also be related to fears of cancer recurrence. Although a person with cancer may deny such fears, he may actually be suppressing them. If a patient's suspicions of a recurrence are confirmed, the resulting emotional distress may be greater than the distress he felt at the time of initial diagnosis. Anorexia is one of the emotional reactions that can be expected when survival becomes a source of concern (9).

The combination of physical and psychological pressures can have very undesirable effects upon appetite. Pain or intense physical discomfort, along with hospitalization and unsuccessful therapeutic measures, can all interfere with the ability to enjoy food.

Anorexia Related to Treatment

When chemotherapy, radiotherapy, or gastrointestinal tract disease prevents a patient from eating, hyperalimentation is available for nutritional support. A patient receiving hyperalimentation for an extended period of time may become psychologically dependent upon it and experience apprehension before, during, or after its discontinuance. Gradual adjustment is suggested for patients who are uneasy about discontinuing hyperalimentation (9).

The psychological relationship of cancer chemotherapy to food cannot be overlooked. A patient anticipating the nausea as a result of chemotherapy may experience psychogenic vomiting; he may vomit before arriving at the clinic or when the needle is inserted. The undesirable effects of the therapy upon appetite are often intensified when the patient is nauseated before the drug is injected (19).

The influence of therapy-related nausea upon the acceptance of particular foods is illustrated by an experiment performed in Seattle on three groups of children. One group of children was given a particular flavor of ice cream just before treatment with toxic drugs. A control group to whom the ice cream was offered received no chemotherapy. Another control group receiving chemotherapy was not offered the ice cream before treatment. Of the three groups, the group receiving chemotherapy after eating the ice cream was the most likely to refuse it when it was offered again (19).

The fact that anorexia appears to be caused by conditioned aversion suggests that appropriate conditioning could be attempted to reverse food dislikes. However, metabolic factors may interfere with the effectiveness of this psychological approach (5).

Anorexia Related to Disease

Anxiety is a problem with which physicians become familiar in cancer patients. It indicates the involvement of the patient's mind in the deterioration of his metabolic functions and the chronic nature of his disease (4).

An assumption is commonly made that cancer patients are depressed. Holland et al. (9) reported on 97 cancer patients who were assessed for physical and non-physical symptoms of depression. Scores were low for such non-physical symptoms as feelings of worthlessness, loss of self-esteem, and pessimism, but were high for physical symptoms such as anorexia, weight loss, and insomnia. The conclusion that physical symptoms of depression do not necessarily indicate clinical depression in cancer patients is based on the following factors. First, the physical symptoms of depression on which cancer patients received high scores are the same as the symptoms of advanced cancer and may reflect physical illness. Second, in cancer patients anorexia and cachexia were associated only with physical symptoms of depression, not with non-physical symptoms such as guilt or feelings of worthlessness. Finally, tricyclic antidepressants were less effective in cancer patients than in patients with psychotic depression.

Since the cancer patient's anorexia is often a somatic symptom rather than an indicator of depression, one might not expect psychological methods to be influential in stimulating appetite. However, there is evidence that such psychological aspects of nutrition as encouragement with eating and arranging for social interaction at meals have value, and should not be overlooked (8,18).

CONCLUSIONS

We need a more adequate understanding of the causes of anorexia in neoplastic disease. To better understand the reasons for a loss of appetite, we need a more thorough understanding of both the normal regulation of food intake and the abnormalities that occur with a malignancy.

There is convincing evidence that nutritional support of the patient improves his ability to tolerate the side effects of various forms of treatment. While nutritional therapy by itself may not significantly prolong life, it can improve the quality of life.

Although the most effective way to improve the appetite of the cancer patient is to control the disease, efforts to increase food intake are recommended even when anorexia prevents food from being pleasurable. The needs and preferences of each patient should be considered in nutritional management.

REFERENCES

1. Berstein, I. L. (1978): Learned taste aversions in children receiving chemotherapy. *Science,* 200:130–132.
2. Brennan, M. F. (1977): Uncomplicated starvation versus cancer cachexia. *Cancer Res.,* 37:2359–2364.
3. Carson, J. S., and Gormican, A. (1977): Taste acuity and food attitudes of selected patients with cancer. *J. Am. Diet. Assoc.,* 70:361–365.
4. Costa, G. (1973): Cachexia and the systemic effects of tumors. In: *Cancer Medicine,* edited by J. F. Holland and E. Frei, pp. 1035–1043. Lea and Febiger, Philadelphia.
5. DeWys, W. D. (1970): Working conference on anorexia and cachexia of neoplastic disease. *Cancer Res.,* 30:2816–2818.

6. DeWys, W. D. (1974): Abnormalities of taste as a remote effect of a neoplasm. *Ann. N.Y. Acad. Sci.,* 230:427–434.
7. DeWys, W. D. (1977): Anorexia in cancer patients. *Cancer Res.,* 37:2354–2358.
8. Hegedus, A., and Pelham, M. (1975): Dietetics in a cancer hospital. *J. Am. Diet. Assoc.,* 67:235–240.
9. Holland, J. C. B., Rowland, J., and Plumb, M. (1977): Psychological aspects of anorexia in cancer patients. *Cancer Res.,* 37:2425–2428.
10. Morrison, S. D. (1975): Origins of nutritional imbalance in cancer. *Cancer Res.,* 35:3339–3342.
11. Morrison, S. D. (1976): Generation and compensation of the cancer cachectic process by spontaneous modification of feeding behavior. *Cancer Res.,* 36:228–233.
12. Morrison, S. D. (1978): Origins of anorexia in neoplastic disease. *Am. J. Clin. Nutr.,* 31:1104–1107.
13. Shils, M. E. (1973): Nutrition and neoplasia. In: *Modern Nutrition in Health and Disease,* edited by R. S. Goodhart and M. E. Shils, pp. 981–996. Lea and Febiger, Philadelphia.
14. Theologides, A. (1972): Pathogenesis of cachexia in cancer: A review and a hypothesis. *Cancer,* 29:484–488.
15. Theologides, A. (1974): The anorexia-cachexia syndrome: A new hypothesis. *Ann. N.Y. Acad. Sci.,* 230:14–22.
16. Theologides, A. (1976): Anorexia-producing intermediary metabolites. *Am. J. Clin. Nutr.,* 29:552–558.
17. Theologides, A. (1976): Why cancer patients have anorexia. *Geriatrics,* 31:69–71.
18. Theologides, A. (1977): Nutritional management of the patient with advanced cancer. *Postgrad. Med.,* 61:97–101.
19. van Eys, J. (1978): Nutrition and cancer in children. *Cancer Bull.,* 30:93–97.

Nutritional Management of the Cancer Patient, edited by J. Wollard.
Raven Press, New York © 1979.

Dietary Management of the Colostomy/Ileostomy Patient

Debra S. Dees and Carol A. Stitt

Department of Nutrition and Food Service, The University of Texas System Cancer Center M. D. Anderson Hospital and Tumor Institute, Houston, Texas 77030

In 1977 it was estimated that there would be approximately 101,000 new cases of colon and/or rectum cancer (1). Surgical resection with the resulting construction of a colostomy or ileostomy is a common method of treatment for this type of cancer. Many of the common problems experienced by ostomy patients can be avoided through proper dietary management.

This chapter gives a general overview of the physiology, nutritional implications, and dietary guidelines to assist the dietitian in the management of the colostomy and ileostomy patient.

ILEOSTOMY

Definition

Ileostomy is the surgical construction of a passageway through the abdominal wall into the ileum (16). Ileostomies were not widely used until the late 1920s and early 1930s. At that time, this surgical procedure was not successful, as many patients were often referred in the later stages of their disease state and in poor physical and/or medical condition. Also, the ileostomy appliances were primitive and inevitable complications related to frequent leakage and skin excoriation occurred.

Physiology

Determination of the placement of the stoma is done prior to surgery. Generally, it is placed in the lower right quadrant, when possible, because of the position of the terminal ileum. It is essential that the stoma be placed on a flat, nonscarred surface, relatively free from irregularities, to avoid postoperative complications with the activities of daily living.

The terminal ileum is extracted through a small circular or oval orifice cut out of the skin. The portion of the ileum that passes through the abdominal wall is considered to be the most vulnerable part of the ileostomy (15). Scar tissue may collect at this point and cause difficulties with passage of contents. The size of the orifice is important, since too small an opening could later cause a stricture and too large an opening may cause a hernia or prolapse.

The ileum proximal to the stoma is sutured to the abdominal wall to avoid small bowel obstruction and gangrene from torsion and volvulus (15). Adequate smooth skin on all sides of the stoma is necessary to alleviate the fear of the ileostomy appliance becoming detached with normal body motions.

The normal color of the stoma is pink to red-orange, and a good indicator of possible ischemia or necrosis is a change in the stoma's color, causing it to appear darker and somewhat bluish (11,12).

The attending physicians and nurses must watch for pulmonary atelectasis, deep venous thrombosis, and infection of either the abdominal or perineal wounds. Oral fluids are generally ordered the first three to four days after initial intravenous feeding. Solid food is introduced gradually to avoid abdominal cramps and nausea (5).

Generally, the ileostomy does not function for several days after surgery, with the exception of small blood discharge from the surgery itself. At first, the daily output is small and it increases with each subsequent day until a plateau is reached. At this time, there is a small contraction in the volume of output and the discharge thickens; this has been called ileostomy adaptation (5). There is evidence to suggest this adaptation is a physiologic response of the small intestine in the gradual assumption of the colon's function, that is, absorption of salt and water. This is thought to be mediated by the mineralocorticoid, aldosterone (5). When regulated, discharges occur at frequent intervals throughout the day, especially after meals. The discharge is pasty to liquid in consistency and high in enzyme content.

Although ileal output varies among patients, some have what is called a "low volume ileostomy" (approximately 500 ml/day) and others a "high volume ileostomy" (approximately 1 liter or more per day), generally a "well-functioning" ileostomy is said to excrete approximately 60 mEq of sodium and 500 ml of water per day (7,8). That is two to three times greater than the feces of normal patients. In situations where the ileum is resected along with the colectomy, a greater amount of drainage usually occurs and special precautions must be taken. However, in a well-functioning ileostomy, with "normal day-to-day living," dietary intake of sodium and water is more than adequate to cover these losses.

The ileostomate does have a significantly lower urine volume and urinary sodium as evidenced by the above-mentioned losses (5). If the ileostomy volume becomes abnormally high, negative balances may occur and other precautions, which will be discussed later in this chapter, must be taken.

Indications

When the colon and rectum are irreparably damaged by inflammatory disease (chronic ulcerative colitis, Crohn's disease, familial polyposis), neoplastic diseases (cancer of colon), ischemic diseases or congenital defects or trauma, ileostomy is deemed the appropriate surgical treatment.

Nutritional Implications

Very little digestion actually takes place in the colon. The fermentative bacteria found in the middle portion do change carbohydrates into carbon dioxide, alcohol, and lactic acid. This is the only means by which our body acts upon cellulose.

No digestive enzymes are secreted in the colon. However, an alkaline fluid helps complete digestion that was begun in the small intestine.

As alluded to earlier, there is a great deal of water and sodium absorbed in the colon which aids in the conservation of body fluids.

Current Findings

Direct studies of body composition reflect that most ileostomates are salt and water depleted. It was found, however, that many were in this state prior to their surgery. Therefore, appropriate nutritional assessment and nutritional build-up with either chemically defined liquid elemental diets or hyperalimentation are appropriate. There is much evidence that suggests hyperalimentation has much value for these patients, both preoperatively and postoperatively (15).

In ileostomates who have not had ileum resection, a 1970 study reports reduced vitamin B_{12} absorption. In this study, the majority of subjects showed borderline values for vitamin B_{12} absorption and 25% had a significant reduction in vitamin B_{12} absorption. The reason for this is unknown, but it has been postulated that a temporary imbalance of microflora in the intestines may be the causative factor (9,15).

Those who have undergone ileum resection do have malabsorption of folic acid and vitamin B_{12}. Regular supplemental vitamin B_{12} injections are necessary for those who have had appreciable ileal resection. These patients do lose a greater amount of fluid and electrolytes and must be encouraged to increase their water and salt intake to help balance their electrolytes.

Studies indicate that in well-functioning ileostomies the quantity of substances excreted is not sufficient to cause clinically apparent deficiencies (with the exception of the above-mentioned water, sodium and vitamin B_{12}), and that good dietary principles are the only necessary guidelines (15).

All ileostomy patients experience occasional episodes of diarrhea as a result of emotional stress, acute infectious gastroenteritis, or dietary indiscretion. In such instances, not only water and salt intake should be encouraged, but also foods high in potassium. There are commercially prepared fluids available that contain electrolytes and glucose (Gatorade, Sportade, Bulldog Punch, Olympade), but their use should be approved by a physician.

Volume output appears to have little relation to any particular foods or fluid consumed, but diets low in sodium or consisting entirely of liquids (chemically defined elemental diets) tend to decrease the output (6). The output, as a result of these two modifications, rarely falls below 40% of the normal output (5).

Complaints of gas and malodorous stools are common among ileostomates. Excessive gas, which is no more common in ileostomates than normal subjects, is generally the result of air ingested during breathing, rapid eating and talking, gum chewing, drinking carbonated beverages, smoking, or anxiety. Certain foods are gas-producing and may need to be eliminated from the diet (see the end of this chapter). These may, however, affect each person differently.

Malodorous stools are usually diet-related and are thought to be due to bacteria acting on particular foods, producing methane, mercaptans, and hydrogen sulfide (15). Some medications (e.g., antibiotics), and vitamin preparations may have the same effect.

Occasionally, excessive weight gain becomes a problem postoperatively (11,15). This usually results from the ileostomate's ability to tolerate more foods that were denied him or were intolerable preoperatively. An appropriate weight reduction regimen should be developed if the problem arises.

Complications

As previously indicated, most ileostomates have occasional diarrhea. However, when it becomes persistent this should trigger an alarm to the patient as well as medical personnel. There are four etiologic factors generally associated with this diarrhea: partial intestinal obstruction, recurrent granulomatous disease, intraabdominal sepsis, and resection of the terminal ileum (5).

Partial intestinal obstruction may arise as a result of ileostomy stenosis, where the bowel becomes dilated just proximal to the stoma, or it may occur as a result of the intestine being compressed by an abnormal band or adhesion. The latter is the most common cause and becomes indicative with the onset of abdominal cramps.

The precise mechanisms for recurrent granulomatous disease have not been identified, but are thought to be similar to the altered water and electrolyte balance as in inflammatory bowel disease (5).

Any patient who has had an ileostomy as a result of Crohn's disease has a strong possibility of developing intraabdominal sepsis. Initially, the patient experiences 'colicky' abdominal pain, borborygmi, and looseness of the ileostomy. Later, the ileostomate consistently has a high volume output that is difficult to control by medicine and, thus, is often resolved through further excisional surgery (5).

As indicated previously, if a significant amount of the ileum is resected at the time of the ileostomy, volume output tends to be unusually high, along with higher sodium and potassium output. In the majority of these patients, medical management is successful. A 1974 study demonstrated that codeine phosphate was the most effective of the three therapeutic agents (codeine phosphate, Lomotil, and Isogel) (13). The codeine phosphate along with additional sodium intake is generally successful in the treatment of this condition (3).

As with any patient experiencing diarrhea, electrolyte and water imbalance must be suspected. In the ileostomy patient, dehydration is normally concomitant with sodium depletion. When the urinary sodium falls below 10 mEq per day and urine volume below 600 ml, the patient is said to have sodium depletion (5). This, along with water, must be replaced orally or intravenously, depending on the severity of the diarrhea.

When oral replacement is appropriate, the patient may be encouraged to drink one 8-ounce glass of any of the following: water with one-half teaspoon salt or bicarbonate of soda, orange juice, tea, cola, or bouillon, and commercial drinks prepared for athletes (Gatorade, Sportade, etc.) (11). However, the physician should be alerted of symptoms and the choice of replacement ratified.

Obstruction is probably one of the most feared complications of ileostomy patients and may occur for a variety of reasons. Not only are the symptoms distressing to the patient (cramps, vomiting, abdominal distention, and virtually total cessation of output) but also immediate medical attention is necessary to monitor dehydration and, more importantly, to prevent necrosis of the bowel itself. Necrosis occurs as a result of either impairment or detainment of the local blood supply and is usually secondary to edema. Four general causes of obstruction are: dysfunction and stenosis, food blockage, adhesions, and volvulus (15).

Food blockage may occur as a result of the food itself or the condition of the bowel. Scar tissue may collect over a period of time and foods that were initially tolerated by the patient may cause difficulties to the point of obstruction at a later time. Often the offending food is of vegetable origin or poorly digestible, such as tough 'stringy' meats and foods high in fiber, as well as foods that are simply not masticated well by a fast eater. Treatment in this particular complication begins with prevention, that is, proper forewarning of such foods and eating habits by the dietitian.

Adhesions impart the same symptoms of food blockage. However, the obstruction is located several inches proximal to the ileostomy outlet. These are often amended successfully through medical treatment, but, sometimes require surgery.

Volvulus is due to torsion of the bowel around a fixed point and frequently occurs where the ileostomy exits from the abdomen. This rapidly jeopardizes the intestinal blood supply and leads to ischemic necrosis and the loss of the majority of the remaining bowel (15).

Postileostomy ileitis occurs in a small percentage of patients, mainly those patients who received the ileostomy as a result of granulomatous or ulcerative colitis. In acute ileitis or 'back wash,' the terminal ileum is superficially inflamed. It is often resolved without the removal of the inflamed ileum, but hemorrhage and diarrhea may occur until it is resolved (15).

A recurrence of regional enteritis is implied with chronic postileostomy ileitis. It may be relatively benign, with an increase in volume output, or produce severe complications (fistulization, peri-ileostomy abscess formation, severe diarrhea, retraction of stoma, and intermittent obstruction). A further loss of absorptive surface is probable whether from the disease itself or the removal of an additional portion of the ileum. In such cases, severe diarrhea and electrolyte problems arise, and the ability to absorb bile salts and vitamin B_{12} is reduced. Treatment is the same as if it occurred prior to the ileostomy.

There is some evidence indicating that those with a greater ileostomy discharge have a higher risk of forming urinary stones. In 1969, a study concluded that the ileostomy patient has a urinary composition that favors uric acid precipitation and, thus, has a greater risk of developing uric acid stones. However, the frequency of development differs from one country to another (2).

It is now known that the loss of an appreciable portion of the terminal ileum has an effect on the enterohepatic circulation of bile acids. Thus, those ileostomates who have had appreciable ileal resections are thought to have a higher risk of developing cholelithiasis (5). A diet restricted in fat may be appropriate if cholecystitis or cholelithiasis occurs.

Other complications that may occur are those of a mechanical nature, that is, skin irritation and ulceration, stomal ulceration and nodules, retraction, prolapse, fistulas, and perineal healing.

Innovations

In 1968, a Swedish surgeon developed an alternate method for the storage of ileal contents, an internal ileal pouch (10). No external appliance is necessary; the patient simply wears a pad over the stoma and periodically inserts a catheter to drain the contents (4). This surgery is complicated and hasn't been completely tested. Thus, only a few large medical centers in the United States have performed this surgical procedure. The advantage of such treatment is that it relieves a lot of the restrictions on physical activity and lessens the emotional adjustment. However, the disadvantages are the skin irritations resulting from more direct exposure with ileal content and a stricter dietary regimen. All foods must be broken down by the time they reach the stoma to pass through the lumen of a catheter. Corn, celery, and nuts are three of the more common problem foods.

COLOSTOMY

Definition

The word colostomy is derived from two Greek words: "colon" (the large bowel) and "stoma" (mouth) (18). A colostomy is the surgical formation of an artificial anus in the mid-abdomen, usually below the waist. The opening may involve different parts of the colon depending on the location of the diseased area: transverse colostomy, ascending colostomy, or sigmoid colostomy. The diseased part of the colon along with the rectum is removed and the stump of the remaining colon is brought forward to the surface of the abdomen.

Physiology

The colon or large intestine is approximately 5 to 6 feet long and 2½ inches in diameter. It is composed of the following sections: the ascending colon, the transverse colon, the descending colon, the sigmoid colon, and the rectum. The rectum consists of the last 7 or 8 inches of the intestine, the terminal inch of which is called the anal canal. The opening of this canal to the outside of the body is called the anus. The main functions of the colon are absorption of water from the fecal mass, storage, and the eventual elimination of these waste products from the body through the anus.

Indications

Some conditions that may necessitate a colostomy are cancer of the rectum or part of the colon, bowel obstruction resulting from tumor spread, and radiation proctitis with fistula or stricture.

Nutritional Implications

The length of the remaining colon determines the consistency or frequency of the output from a colostomy. The patient with a transverse colostomy will experience a more frequent and liquid output since it is closer to the ileocecal valve. There is also a much smaller area allowed for storage of waste material. The patient with a sigmoid colostomy will experience more solid output since this section of the colon is located in the lower digestive tract (12).

Odor and flatus are two problems the colostomy patient has to deal with. Colostomy odor may be caused by taking certain oral medications, by the ingestion of certain foods, and by the action of bacteria on waste material in the colon. Flatus or gas is a common problem that is both embarrassing and a major reason why a colostomate avoids social situations. There is no way to stop gas formation, but one can do certain things to control it. The person with a colostomy can try to avoid swallowing air, which can lead to gas formation, and he can avoid gas-forming foods in his diet (3,4,14,17).

Constipation is another problem the colostomy patient may

experience (11). Often, just increasing one's fluid intake will prove to be beneficial in controlling this problem. Foods with a mild laxative effect may be added to the diet. If these suggestions are ineffective, the colostomy patient should consult a physician. A laxative can be very dangerous for a colostomy patient and no drugs should be taken without a physician's consent.

Diarrhea can hit the colostomy patient just as it does anyone else. It can be caused by food poisoning, intestinal flu, cobalt treatments, and certain drugs such as types of antibiotics and chemotherapeutic agents (4). The patient should consult his physician if he is experiencing acute diarrhea. There are some foods that may provide relief in cases of mild diarrhea. These will be discussed later in this chapter.

Dietary Guidelines

At M. D. Anderson Hospital the following guidelines are used for the ostomy patient:

1. Select foods carefully at first, then add new foods *one at a time*. Patients should not be afraid to experiment.

2. Keep a record of foods that are bothersome and what effects they have. Although a food may disagree with the patient the first time he tries it, after a few weeks it may not present a problem.

3. Eat regularly. Skipping meals will not eliminate gas, but may actually increase it.

4. Eat in a pleasant, relaxed atmosphere. Remember: emotional upsets, tension, or travel may cause bowel problems even with foods the patient is accustomed to.

5. Chew foods slowly and thoroughly. Chew with a closed mouth, and avoid excessive talking while eating; swallowed air may increase gas.

6. If the patient has been following another special diet, the physician or dietitian should be notified so the patient's diet may be combined with ostomy management.

7. Eat in an upright position if possible, rather than lying down.

The following food lists have been compiled and utilized at M. D. Anderson Hospital in the treatment of ostomy patients. These foods have been found to cause problems in some patients, but individual tolerance will vary.

Gas-producing foods:
1. Dried beans and peas
2. Vegetables of the cabbage family (broccoli, Brussels sprouts, cabbage, cauliflower)
3. Asparagus
4. Sweet potatoes
5. Onions
6. Eggs
7. Fish
8. Certain cheeses (Roquefort, Brie, and other strong cheeses)
9. Milk
10. Melons
11. Nuts
12. Sugar, sweets, sweetened drinks
13. Beer

High fiber foods that may cause irritation:
1. Foods with seeds, hard to digest kernels, or cellulose
2. Some raw fruits such as oranges, apples, strawberries
3. Some raw vegetables such as coleslaw, salad greens, celery
4. Some cooked vegetables such as spinach, green beans, corn
5. Popcorn
6. Nuts
7. Coconut
8. Highly seasoned foods
9. Tomatoes

Foods that may contribute to diarrhea:
1. Green leafy vegetables

2. Broccoli
3. Beans
4. Raw fruits
5. Highly seasoned foods
6. Beer

Foods that may help control diarrhea:

1. Bananas
2. Applesauce
3. Rice
4. Tapioca
5. Creamy peanut butter

To help control mild constipation:

1. Increase fluids
2. Increase fruit juices
3. Increase cooked fruits and vegetables

Foods that help reduce odors:

1. Cranberry juice
2. Yogurt
3. Buttermilk

Foods that may produce strong odors:

1. Fish
2. Chicken
3. Eggs
4. Onions

REFERENCES

1. American Cancer Society. (1976): *1977 Cancer Facts and Figures.* American Cancer Society, Inc., New York.
2. Clarke, A. M., and McKenzie, R. G. (1969): Ileostomy and the risk of urinary acid stones. *Lancet,* 2:395–397.
3. Diebler, C. A., and Britton, L. (1978): Dietary tolerance of ostomates. *Et Journal,* Winter: 14, 5:1.
4. Happenie, S. D. (1968): *Colostomy, A Second Change.* Charles C Thomas, Springfield, Illinois.
5. Hill, G. L. (1976): *Ileostomy: Surgery, Physiology, and Management.* Grune and Stratton, New York.

6. Hill, G. L., Mair, W. S. J., Edwards, J. P., Morgan, D. B., and Goligher, J. C. (1975): Effect of chemically defined liquid elemental diet on composition and volume of ileal fistula drainage. *Gastroenterology*, 68:676–682.
7. Hill, G. L., Mair, W. S. J., and Goligher, J. C. (1974): Impairment of ileostomy adaptation in patients after ileal resection. *Gut*, 15:982–987.
8. Hill, G. L., Mair, W. S. J., and Goligher, J. C. (1975): Cause and management of high volume output salt depleting ileostomy. *Br. J. Surg.*, 62:720–726.
9. Hulten, L., Kewenter, J., Persson, E., and Ahren, C. (1970): Vitamin B_{12} absorption in ileostomy patients after operation for ulcerative colitis. *Scand. J. Gastroenterol.*, 5:113–116.
10. Koch, N. G. (1969): Intra-abdominal reservoir in patients with permanent ileostomy. *Arch. Surg.* 99:223.
11. Mahoney, J. M. (1976): *Guide to Ostomy Nursing Care*. Little, Brown, and Company, Boston.
12. Mahoney, J. M. (1978): What you should know about ostomies. *Nursing*, 8 (May): 74–84.
13. Newton, C. R. (1973): The effect of codeine perosphate, lomotil and isogel on ileostomy function. *Gut*, 14:424–425.
14. Rowbotham, J. L. (1971): Colostomy problems-dietary and colostomy management. *Cancer*, 28:219–238.
15. Sparberg, M. D., and Marshall, N. (1971): *Ileostomy Care*. Charles C Thomas, Springfield, Illinois.
16. Thomas, M. D., and Clayton, L., editors (1973): *Taber's Cyclopedic Medical Dictionary*. F. A. Davis Company, Philadelphia.
17. Vukovich, V. C., and Grubb, R. D. (1973): *Care of the Ostomy Patient*. C. V. Mosby Company, St. Louis.
18. Walker, F. C. (1976): *Modern Stoma Care*. Churchill Livingstone, Edinburgh.

Nutritional Management of the Cancer Patient, edited by J. Wollard.
Raven Press, New York © 1979.

Lactose Malabsorption

Kay Martin

Department of Nutrition and Food Service, The University of Texas System Cancer Center M. D. Anderson Hospital and Tumor Institute, Houston, Texas 77030

Lactose malabsorption is a critical factor to consider when prescribing nutritional therapy for the cancer patient. The initial nutritional interview should try to determine if lactose malabsorption exists before treatment is begun. Thereafter, an ongoing case review is imperative to identify any therapy-induced lactase deficiency, and to halt its effects. Without the hydrolyzing effect of lactase, lactose will not be absorbed and diarrhea can result. The consequent loss of undigested carbohydrate along with fat, protein, fluid, and electrolytes is a significant consideration when planning to meet the nutritional needs of the cancer patient.

Lactose, a disaccharide (beta-galactoside), is found predominantly in milk and milk products. Each lactose molecule, after being ingested, is hydrolyzed to one molecule each of glucose and galactose. Part of the resulting glucose may be used locally in the intestine for energy, while the remaining glucose and galactose are absorbed into the intestinal epithelial cells.

There are three known enzymes with beta-galactosidase activity, but only one is thought to be responsible for the hydrolysis of lactose. This is "neutral lactase," or lactase, and appears to work optimally at a pH of 5.5 to 6 (9). The enzyme is formed in the microvilli (brush border) of the intestinal epithelial cells, with highest specific activity in the jejunum (9).

Occasionally, one of several lactase deficiency syndromes

prevents the formation of lactase. When this occurs, a small amount of the unhydrolyzed lactose may be absorbed by passive diffusion into the urine. The remaining unabsorbed lactose attracts water and sodium chloride into the lumen of the intestine. This osmotic process continues until the contents of the intestine and the extracellular fluid reach an equilibrium. The increased fluid content in the intestine acts as a stimulus to peristalsis, decreasing transit time. As the undigested lactose moves rapidly through the gastrointestinal tract, colonic bacteria metabolize a portion to hydrogen gas, acetic acid, and lactic acid. The result is a presentation of watery, fermentative diarrhea, accompanied by flatulence and cramping. Occasionally, nausea and even vomiting may occur. The significant factor here is the loss of undigested carbohydrate and other nutrients, due to the increased intestinal motility and resulting malabsorption. If these conditions persist, a diagnosis of malnutrition is inevitable.

TYPES OF LACTOSE MALABSORPTION

Research documents the existence of several different types of lactose malabsorption: congenital, secondary, primary, and relative (3–6). Congenital lactose malabsorption is an extremely rare condition in which there is a complete absence of lactase. Symptoms begin immediately following birth, soon after milk feedings are begun. Symptoms are relieved when lactose-free feedings are given and reappear when the patient is again given lactose. Because the nutritional prescription for the cancer patient often includes numerous milk-based nutritional supplements, the dietitian's nutritional interview should search for this type of lactose malabsorption in the patient's history.

Secondary lactose malabsorption is a more common form. It is presumed that, in these cases, a primary cause (such as bacteria, malnutrition, toxin, or a drug) leads to intestinal mucosal damage accompanied by secondary loss of lactase (see Table 1). One primary causative factor, malnutrition, is highly prevalent in the cancer patient and leads to flattening and broadening

TABLE 1. *Secondary lactose malabsorption syndromes*[a]

Associated with:
1. Infectious or nonspecific diarrhea in infancy
2. Malnutrition in infancy
3. Gluten-induced enteropathy
4. Tropical sprue
5. Cystic fibrosis
6. Ulcerative colitis, regional enteritis, blind loop syndromes
7. Gastrectomy or extensive resection of the small intestine
8. *Giardia lamblia* infestation
9. Beta-lipoprotein deficiency
10. Immunologic deficiency syndromes
11. Necrotizing enterocolitis
12. Drugs
    A. Neomycin
    B. Colchicine
    C. Birth control pills

[a] Modified from ref. 9, with permission.

of the intestinal villi. Both membrane surface and disaccharidase activity are decreased, leading to malabsorption.

All forms of cancer treatment, i.e., surgery, drugs, radiation, etc., can result in a secondary lactose malabsorption. Secondary lactose malabsorption syndromes have been observed following gastrectomy and extensive resection of the small intestine (7). Since lactase production is located in the vulnerable intestinal epithelial cells, it may be especially devastated by radiation and chemotherapeutic agents, which particularly affect cells with a high rate of regeneration.

Primary lactose malabsorption, selective lactose malabsorption, acquired lactase deficiency, constitutional hypolactasia, or ontogenetic lactose malabsorption are all terms used to identify the syndrome present in persons who have reached the age where lactase activity is low—usually anyone over the age of 1½ to 3 years (see Fig. 1). Lactase concentrations remain at a high level throughout adulthood in only a few population groups, including most northern European and white American ethnic groups and

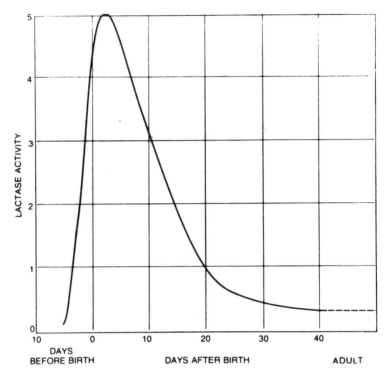

FIG. 1. Lactase is present in mammals other than man, and in most humans, in the fetus before birth, and in infancy. The general shape of the curve of enzyme activity, shown here for rats, is about the same for all species. Enzyme activity, given here in relative units, is determined by measuring glucose release from intestinal tissue in the presence of lactose.

East African Nilotic Negroes (9). The exact mechanism involved in the appearance and disappearance of lactase is not known, but it is believed to be an evolutionary and genetic process, possibly a throwback to primitive man's decreased consumption of milk after weaning. In any case, the nutritional counselor must be attentive to the cancer patient's racial and ethnic identity.

One other form of lactose malabsorption has been identified: relative lactose malabsorption, defined as "the inability to completely utilize a large load of lactose" (6). It is thought that relative lactose malabsorption may be present in a majority of adults. It may occur especially in adult patients who ingest large quantities of milk, for example, ulcer patients, pregnant women, or patients who are tube fed with a milk-based formula. This factor is another to consider when prescribing the type and quantity of nutritional supplement to be utilized by the cancer patient.

CONFIRMATION OF LACTOSE MALABSORPTION

To positively confirm lactose malabsorption one must make use of laboratory techniques, i.e., lactose loading, intestinal biopsy, fecal pH, and breath hydrogen analysis. Lactose loading, similar to the glucose tolerance test, utilizes the administration of megadoses of lactose to the fasting patient. If blood glucose levels increase less than 20 mg/100 m, and symptoms occur, the diagnosis is positive for lactose malabsorption.

Intestinal biopsy is considered the most reliable method for establishing a diagnosis of lactose malabsorption (9). In this test, a small tube is channeled into the small intestine, and a portion of the lining is retrieved to measure the enzyme level. The so-called "normal" range of lactase activity varies greatly, but the lower limit for normal activity is from 0.5 to 2.0 units per gram of mucosa.

The fecal pH test for lactose malabsorption is useful only for screening children. If the child's fecal pH measures less than 6, he is considered to be intolerant of lactose, since acid stools are the result of bacterial metabolism of lactose to lactic and acetic acids. This test is not useful for adults, as adult stools normally have an acid pH, nor is it valid for patients taking antibiotics.

Breath hydrogen analysis after ingestion of lactose may be used to identify lactose malabsorbers. Samples of expired air are analyzed by gas chromatography, to determine the proportion of hydrogen. Exhaled hydrogen is derived from intestinal hydrogen, which in turn is derived from the fermentation of undigested lactose. The amount of hydrogen in the exhaled air is greater in lactose malabsorbers than in lactose absorbers.

ROLE OF THE DIETITIAN IN COMBATING LACTOSE MALABSORPTION

Because of the expense and time involved, the tests described above are rarely performed. The dietitian, through careful patient interviewing, is often the first member of the medical team to perceive the presence of lactose malabsorption. The patient who complains of gas, indigestion, diarrhea, or vague abdominal pain 30 to 60 min after ingesting milk or milk products may be suspected as a lactose malabsorber. Further clues suggesting this syndrome can be a family history of milk intolerance, membership in a high-prevalence group, or the recent consumption of more lactose-containing products than usual. When a diagnosis of lactose intolerance is made, a lactose-free, restricted-residue diet may be indicated, with attention given to sodium, potassium, and fluid intake. Individualization of the diet is of the utmost importance. If the patient is counseled about the amount of lactose that foods contain, he is often able to determine his own tolerance.

Some general guidelines that might be helpful to a patient are:

1. Drink liquids between meals, rather than with meals, to decrease osmotic activity in the gut.

2. Eat foods at room temperature, rather than very cold or very hot, to avoid rapid transit time of food in the intestine.

3. Eat smaller amounts of food more frequently, to enhance absorption.

4. Eat foods in which the lactose has been partially or completely broken down by the organisms they contain.

5. Utilize low-lactose, lactose-reducing, or lactose-free products whenever nutritional build-up is essential.

Although current literature advocates the use of a restricted-residue diet in dealing with diarrhea, there have been some reports of studies in which the inclusion of small amounts of bran in the diet appears to slow down intestinal transit time, thus helping to alleviate diarrhea (8).

Lactose malabsorption may present a problem for the cancer patient. However, given knowledge of its causes and physiology, careful patient monitoring, and counseling, the patient and dietitian can deal successfully with this problem.

REFERENCES

1. Bayless, T. M., and Rosensweig, N. S. (1967): Topics in clinical medicine. Incidence and implications of lactase deficiency and milk intolerance in white and Negro populations. *Johns Hopkins Med. J.,* 121:54.
2. Boellner, S. W., Beard, A. G., and Panos, T. C. (1965): Impairment of intestinal hydrolysis of lactose in newborn infants. *Pediatrics,* 36:542.
3. Calloway, D. J., Murphy, E. L., and Baner, D. (1969): Determination of lactose intolerance by breath analysis. *Am. J. Dig. Dis.,* 14:811.
4. Christopher, N. L., and Bayless, T. M. (1971): Role of small bowel and colon in lactose-induced diarrhea. *Gastroenterol.,* 60:845.
5. Gray, G. M., and Santiago, N. A. (1969): Intestinal β-galactosidases. I. Separation and characterization of three enzymes in normal human intestine. *J. Clin. Invest.,* 48:716.
6. Harvey, R. F., Pomare, E., and Heaton, K. Q. (1973): Effects of increased dietary fiber on intestinal transit. *Lancet,* 1:1278–1280.
7. Herbst, J. J., Sunshine, P., and Kretchmer, N. (1969): Intestinal malabsorption in infancy and childhood. In: *Advances in Pediatrics,* edited by I. Schulman, pp. 11–64. Year Book Medical Publishers, Inc., Chicago.
8. Holzel, A., Schwartz, V., and Sutcliffe, K. W. (1959): Defective lactose absorption causing malnutrition in infancy. *Lancet,* 1:1126.
9. Johnson, J. D., Kretchmer, N., and Simoons, J. F. (1974): Lactose malabsorption, its biology and history. In: *Advances in Pediatrics,* vol. 21, edited by I. Schulman, pp. 197–237. Year Book Medical Publishers, Inc., Chicago.
10. Kretchmer, N. (1972): Lactose and lactase. *Scientific Amer.,* 227:70–78.
11. Lathamm, M. C. (1977): Public health importance of milk intolerance. *Nutrit. News,* 40:13–16.
12. Laws, J. W., and Neale, G. (1966): Radiological diagnosis of disaccharidase deficiency. *Lancet,* 2:139.

13. Launiala, K. (1968): The mechanism of diarrhea in congenital disaccharide malabsorption. *Acta Paediatr. Scand.*, 57:425.
14. Wailike, B. C., and Wailike, J. W. (1977): Relative lactose intolerance. A clinical study of tube-fed patients. *JAMA*, 238:948–951.

Nutritional Management of the Cancer Patient, edited by J. Wollard.
Raven Press, New York © 1979.

Nutritional Management of the Leukemia Patient

Barbara Saunders

Department of Nutrition and Food Service, The University of Texas System Cancer Center M. D. Anderson Hospital and Tumor Institute, Houston, Texas 77030

The nutritional management of the patient with leukemia presents a unique and challenging opportunity for the dietitian. Briefly, leukemia is the neoplastic formation of hematopoietic cells in which maturation and functional capability are impaired. The accumulation of leukemic cells is most prominent in the bone marrow, but may also occur in the lymph nodes, spleen, and other tissues.

LEUKEMIA

Leukemia is actually a group of diseases, with the type of leukemia identified by the type of white cells affected. Lymphocytic leukemia involves cells originating in the lymph nodes, while myelocytic leukemia involves granulocytes, which are cells produced by myeloid (bone marrow) tissues. Both types can be acute or chronic. In acute leukemia, white cells accumulate more rapidly than in the chronic type of disease. The white cells in acute leukemia are large, immature precursors of normal cells, which cannot carry out the infection-combating functions of normal white cells (4,7). Characteristics of the main types of leukemia are listed in Table 1.

Symptoms of leukemia that may aid in diagnosing the disease are anemia (manifested by pallor, malaise, easy fatigability); pneumonia; thrombocytopenia; infections of the skin; bleeding

TABLE 1. *Characteristics of main types of leukemia*[a]

Type	Age/sex incidence	Onset of symptoms	Treatment	Prognosis
Acute lymphocytic leukemia (ALL)	Most commonly 3 to 4 years old. Rare after age 15. Slightly increased among males.	Sudden onset, symptoms rarely present more than 6 weeks prior to diagnosis.	Very responsive to chemotherapy.	5 year survival = 50%. Some indefinite disease-free survivors. Slightly poorer prognosis in adults.
Chronic lymphocytic leukemia (CML)	Most commonly 50 to 70 years old, rare before age 35; increased incidence with age. Excess among males.	Symptoms may not interfere with life of patient for years.	Not very responsive to chemotherapy. Main treatment is to fight infections.	Variable; median survival is 7 years.
Acute myelogenous leukemia (AML)	Most commonly young adults, but nearly equal frequency among all age groups. Slightly increased among males.	Onset of symptoms may be abrupt, but usually a prodromal period of 1 to 6 months.	Similar to ALL, but needs increased chemotherapy (more resistant to treatment).	Untreated median survival = 2 months, treated = 13 months.
Chronic myelogenous leukemia (CML)	Most commonly 30 to 50 years old. Uncommon before age 20. Slightly increased among males.	Usually gradual.	Chemotherapy, splenectomy (for splenic enlargement).	Median survival = 3 to 5 years, but eventually all reach blastic crisis.

[a] From refs. 2, 10, and 13.

(especially common from the nose and gums in acute lympho-cytic leukemia); enlargement of lymph nodes, hepatomegaly and splenomegaly (leading to feeling of early satiety, therefore decreased intake and weight loss); and heat intolerance with profuse sweating (7).

The exact cause of leukemia in humans remains unknown. However, several factors have been identified as possibly con-tributing to the development of the disease. Ionizing radiation is one of these factors. An increased frequency (30 times that of the normal population) of leukemia was found among Japa-nese survivors of Hiroshima (4). Chemical exposure (to ben-zene, for example) is another environmental factor that may predispose one to leukemia. The increased incidence of leukemia among identical twins and siblings has suggested a heredity factor as the cause. There is a marked increase of chronic myelogenous leukemia (CML) among Down's syndrome pa-tients. An abnormality occurs in the 21st and 22nd pair of chromosomes in each disease (4,7). A viral etiology has also been proposed, since viruses (or virus-like particles) have been found in the blood of leukemia patients. It is hypothesized that these RNA-containing viruses may be transmitted by a yet un-known physiological or chemical factor (4,11).

TREATMENT

The aim of the treatment for leukemia is to achieve remission of the disease. Complete remission is the relief from symptoms, with a return to normal amounts of red blood cells, competent white cells, platelets, and as low a number of leukemic cells in the bone marrow, blood, and tissues as possible. At this time, no treatment can permanently arrest the inevitable recurrence of leukemia, because the available means of therapy cannot remove all leukemic cells; the introduction of a single leukemic cell can produce leukemia in laboratory animals (4). The affected tis-sues are throughout the body, so that surgical excision or high dose irradiation cannot effect a complete cure (9). However, in recent years, development of drugs and improvement of total supportive care have helped decrease the suffering and increase the productive life of leukemia patients.

Chemotherapy

Chemotherapy is the most widely used treatment for leukemia. Acute lymphocytic leukemia (ALL) is more sensitive to chemotherapy than the other types, with over 85% of ALL patients achieving complete remission through induction chemotherapy (4,5). Although other types are more resistant, a variety of antineoplastic agents are used singly or in combinations to help achieve remission. Chemotherapeutic agents are discussed in detail in the chapter on chemotherapy; however, some of the agents that are used in the treatment of leukemia and their possible nutritionally-related consequences are summarized in Table 2.

The dietitian must become familiar with the particular drug regimen of the patient to tailor the diet to the patient's needs in relation to his chemotherapy. The patient should be made aware of the possible side effects, and must be taught alternate methods of achieving intake. For example, if methotrexate is to be given, nausea, vomiting, diarrhea, gastrointestinal (GI) ulcers and stomatitis may be anticipated. The diet should, therefore, be altered to include soft, bland, or liquid feedings, depending on the severity of the patient's reactions to the drugs.

Bone Marrow Transplantation

A complex form of therapy that was seldom used in the past, but which is being used increasingly, is bone marrow transplantation. The procedure, reduced to simplest terms, is an attempt to destroy the leukemic marrow and replace it with healthy cells. Marrow transplants may be autologous (taken from the patient himself while in remission and stored) or allo-

TABLE 2. *Chemotherapeutic drugs used in treatment of leukemia*[a]

Drug	Nutritional side effects
L-asparaginase (Elspar)	50% have nausea and vomiting; hypoalbuminemia, hyperglycemia
Busulfan (Myleran®)	Rarely nausea and vomiting; renal damage
Chlorambucil (Leukeran®)	Large doses cause nausea and vomiting
Cyclophosphamide (Cytoxan®)	Possible hemorrhagic cystitis, some stomatitis, nausea and vomiting 3 to 4 hours after dose
Cytosine arabinoside (Ara-C; Cytosar®)	Nausea, vomiting, esophagitis, diarrhea
3-Deazauridine	Animal studies showed vomiting, diarrhea, GI tract atrophy and necrosis
Daunorubicin	Nausea, vomiting, stomatitis, abdominal pain
Mercaptopurine (Purinethol®; 6-MP)	Nausea, vomiting, stomatitis, diarrhea
Methanesulfon-*m*-anisidide (AMSA)	Animal studies showed anorexia, vomiting, diarrhea, weight loss
Methotrexate	Nausea, vomiting, GI ulcerations; nephrotoxic at high doses
Neocarzinostatin	22% have nausea and vomiting; at high doses—acute enterocolitis
Piperazinedione	Nausea and vomiting, usually mild
Prednisone	Increased appetite, Na and fluid retention, K+ loss, hyperglycemia, GI bleeding and ulcers
Rubidazone	Nausea and vomiting, mucositis, acute fever and chills
Thioguanine	Some nausea and vomiting, stomatitis, diarrhea
Vincristine (Oncovin®)	Abdominal colic, diarrhea or severe constipation, nausea, vomiting

[a] From Department of Pharmaceutical Services, M. D. Anderson Hospital and Tumor Institute; and ref. 8.

$\longrightarrow$

genic (from a relative or sibling). The recipient is given high doses of chemotherapy and/or total body irradiation before the transplant, in an effort to reduce the number of leukemic cells to a minimum, as well as to reduce the possibility of rejection of an allogenic graft. Severe marrow depression results, and the patient must therefore be "rescued" by the bone marrow transplant (4,16).

Side effects of total body irradiation are listed in Table 3. Delayed effects may include hyperpigmentation, peeling of the skin, cataracts, sterility, growth retardation, and liver and kidney damage (15). I have also observed decreased salivary activity and altered taste acuity in patients following total body irradiation.

After total body irradiation, the actual transplant is done, wherein 500 to 700 ml of marrow are infused into the recipient. The marrow migrates from the bloodstream to the marrow spaces of the bones. Because the side effects of high-dose chemotherapy and total body irradiation include severe mucositis, decreased salivary gland activity, possible malabsorption, and commonly, infections of the mouth and throat, the patient cannot and is not expected to maintain adequate oral intake. In addition to oral intake of a diet-as-tolerated, intravenous hyperalimentation (IVH) is begun immediately in order to maintain good nutritional support.

TABLE 3. *Total body irradiation side effects*[a]

	Occurs	Subsides
Nausea and vomiting	Within few hours	Within 24 hr
Alopecia	Within 2 weeks	Within several months
Parotitis, pancreatitis	Within 24 to 72 hr	Within 24 to 72 hr
Diarrhea	Within few hours	Within few days
Fever	Within few hours	Within 24 hr
Erythema	During RX	Within 48 to 72 hr
Mucositis	Within several days	Within weeks

[a] From ref. 15.

The graft-versus-host (GVH) reaction is the primary obstacle to the use of allogenic transplants. GVH occurs if the grafted (donor) cells recognize the recipient as "foreign," leading to a serious immunological attack. GVH affects 70% of allogenic transplants. The target organs of the reaction are the skin, GI tract and liver. Symptoms include skin rashes and infection, anorexia, nausea, vomiting, diarrhea, hepatomegaly, increased bilirubin, and changes in liver enzymes. The fever (and wasting) produced by GVH lead to increased chances of infection and mortality (9,11,12).

Immunotherapy

Immunotherapy is another form of therapy that, although still under investigation, is showing favorable results. As a recognized treatment for cancer, it is newer than surgery, chemotherapy, or radiation therapy. The immune response begins when an antigen (foreign chemical, bacteria, or virus) reacts with an immunocompetent host cell (antibody or cell that is specific for one antigen). Upon second challenge, the host recognizes the antigen and produces increased concentrations of antibodies. It is theorized that the body produces malignant cells constantly, but that the immune system normally recognizes and destroys them (10,13,14). This theory is supported by studies with animals and humans that have demonstrated antigens specific to cancer. Other clinical observations supporting the theory of immunologic surveillance are: occasional spontaneous regressions, an increased rate of cancer in patients with immunological defects (congenital or acquired, as with renal transplants), and lack of development of tumors in patients who have positive cancer cells in washings (2,14). Failure of the body's defense system against cancer may be caused by antigenically different new tumor cells that the body does not recognize as foreign due to low antigenicity, environmental causes, lymphocyte production deficiencies, or congenital deficiencies (10).

The goal of immunotherapy is to stimulate and use the body's defense mechanisms against cancer. The immune system can handle only a limited number of tumor cells, and is therefore used as an adjunct to surgery, chemotherapy, or radiation, rather than as a primary therapy (1,13,14). Different types of immunotherapy are being used and studied in leukemia patients, as well as in other types of cancer. The ultimate value of immunotherapy will require years to determine.

Active immunotherapy may be specific or non-specific. In the *specific* type of immunotherapy, a certain antigen is used to stimulate a specific host response. The patient is vaccinated with killed, irradiated, or extracts of tumor cells (2,10,14). *Non-specific* immunotherapy uses various noncancer antigens to stimulate the immune system, in general (7,10,11,14). Some examples of agents used include: Bacillus Calmette-Guerin (BCG), Corynebacterium parvulum (*C. parvulum*), 2,4-dinitrochlorobenzene (DNCB), and methanol extracted residue of BCG (MER) (2).

Passive immunotherapy involves the use of antibodies or sensitized cells made outside the host. Lymphocytes, or RNA or transfer factor, may be incubated with tumor cells or tumor-specific antigens, then reintroduced into the host (10,14). Lymphocytes from cured cancer patients may be used to transfer established immunity to the host, or patients with the same blood and tumor types may be cross-injected with living, irradiated tumor tissues. After 10 to 14 days, the leukocytes are transfused back to the donor, hopefully carrying increased immunity to him (2,14). With the aid of passive immunity, which is transient, adoptive immunotherapy may occur as the host subsequently develops his own active immunity (10). Side-effects that may occur during administration of some types of immunotherapy include a flu-like syndrome of chills, fever, malaise, nausea, and body aches (1,12). The dietitian should encourage intake as tolerated during this time, including plenty of fluids and light, frequent feedings.

COMPLICATIONS

The complications of leukemia and those caused by the treatment of the disease are often devastating. As leukemic cells increase and invade the bone marrow, production of normal red and white cells is decreased, leading to anemia, infection, or hemorrhage (4,6). Chemotherapeutic agents may compound these problems, since normal cells are compromised in the process of destroying leukemic cells. Anemia is due to increased destruction of red blood cells or blood loss and is treated with transfusions. Hemorrhaging is due to low platelet levels (3). Bleeding of the oral mucosa, GI tract, nose, skin, kidneys, bladder, lungs, optic fundi, or brain may occur (13). Infections may be due to a decrease in normal white blood cells, or impairment of immune response secondary to chemotherapy. Hemorrhage is treated with platelet transfusions, and white cell transfusions and antibiotics are used to combat infection (3,4, 13). It has been estimated that infection and hemorrhage account for 80% of the immediate causes of death in leukemia patients (4).

ROLE OF THE DIETITIAN

Although multiple factors are involved, good nutritional status is a positive factor in the patient's ability to tolerate therapy and resist infections. All efforts should be made to prevent weight loss. Constant encouragement and supplementation with commercial products, foods, or cool, soothing liquids are needed. Patients are encouraged to take advantage of periods between treatments to regain any lost nutritional ground. Unless contraindicated, IVH should be used in patients who are in poor nutritional status at initiation of therapy, or who cannot maintain oral intake. The dietitian's role in weaning the patient from IVH once his disease is stable or treatment is stopped is extremely important. She must follow the patient closely and encourage intake of light, frequent feedings at first, then gradually increase intake. Because platelet counts may be reduced, the danger of trauma to the nasal, esophageal, or gastric mucosa, and resultant hemorrhage contraindicates the insertion of a tube in many cases for the leukemia patient. Visitation at mealtimes (at least once per day) is a must in order to tailor the patient's diet to his frequently changing condition. Rounds with the health care team (including physicians, nurses, pharmacist, social workers, and dental oncologist) serve as an important means of communication and formulation of a total health care plan. The dietitian should follow patients' weights and caloric intakes, and suggest alternate methods of feeding if the patient cannot maintain sufficient intake. Calorie counts are a valuable tool for determining a patient's true intake. Calorie counts can also be used as reinforcement if the patient is given a "goal" (desired caloric level) and praised as he comes nearer to his desired goal each day.

It is not uncommon for the leukemia patient to be hospitalized for several weeks or even months. Even the most varied hospital menu may become monotonous to these patients. Flexibility of the dietary department is invaluable. If possible, the patients should be allowed to request special items. Families may want to bring in favorite foods, which help to eliminate boredom. These foods should, however, be monitored to insure that they are allowed on the patient's diet, are wholesome, and stored properly.

In summary, the leukemia patient's nutritional status is constantly being challenged by the disease itself, as well as by treatment with high-dose chemotherapy, immunotherapy, and/or total body irradiation and bone marrow transplantation. The most important responsibility of the dietitian is to follow the therapy of each patient closely, since his condition may change rapidly, and to adjust his diet accordingly in an effort to maintain optimal nutritional status.

REFERENCES

1. Blast, R. C., Zbar, B., Borsos, T., and Rapp, H. (1974): BCG and cancer. *N. Engl. J. Med.,* 290:1413–1470.
2. Bochow, A. J. (1976): Cancer immunotherapy: What promise does it hold? *Nursing '76,* 6:50–56.
3. Bodey, G. (1970): Supportive care of the cancer patient. *Postgrad. Med.,* 48:203–210.
4. Frei, E., and Freireich, E. (1964): Leukemia. *Sci. Amer.,* 210: 88–96.
5. Freireich, E. (1965): The control of acute leukemia. *Marquette Med. Rev.,* 31:108–110.
6. Freireich, E., Bodey, G., de Jongh, D., and Hersh, E. (1970): Supportive therapeutic measures for patients under treatment for leukemia or lymphoma. In: *Leukemia—Lymphoma,* pp. 275–284. Year Book Medical Publishers, Inc., Chicago.
7. Lichtman, M. A., and Klempeser, M. R. (1974): Leukemia. In: *Clinical Oncology for Medical Students and Physicians,* edited by P. Rubin, pp. 458–470. University of Rochester, New York.
8. Marino, E. B., and Le Blanc, D. H. (1975): Cancer chemotherapy. *Nursing '75,* 5:22–28.
9. Mathe, G., Amiel, J., Schwarzenburg, L., Caltan, A., and Schneider, M. (1973): Treatment of acute leukemia by allogenic bone marrow graft. In: *Progress in Clinical Cancer,* volume III, edited by I. Ariel, pp. 309–319. Grune and Stratton, New York.
10. Moore, G. E. (1973): Clinical aspects of cancer immunity. In: *Progress in Clinical Cancer,* volume V, edited by I. Ariel, pp. 107–120. Grune and Stratton, New York.
11. National Cancer Institute (1976): Progress against leukemia. D.H.E.W. Publication 76–367.
12. Ohnuma, T., and Holland, J. (1977): Nutritional consequences of cancer chemotherapy and immunotherapy. *Cancer Res.,* 37: 2395–2406.
13. Pochedly, C. (1973): *The Child with Leukemia.* Charles C Thomas, Springfield, Illinois.
14. Silverstein, M. J., and Morton, D. L. (1973): Cancer immunotherapy. *Amer. J. Nurs.,* 73:1178–1181.
15. Varricchio, C. G. (1977): Nursing care during total body irradiation. *Amer. J. Nurs.,* 77:1314–1317.
16. Zimmerman, S., Cohen, T., Diekman, R., Calvo, C. L., and Hangsterfer, M. (1977): Bone marrow transplantation. *Amer. J. Nurs.,* 77:1311–1315.

Nutritional Management of the Cancer Patient, edited by J. Wollard.
Raven Press, New York © 1979.

Nutrition in the Pediatric Cancer Patient

Patricia Carter

Department of Nutrition and Food Service, The University of Texas System Cancer Center M. D. Anderson Hospital and Tumor Institute, Houston, Texas 77030

Excluding accidents, cancer is the number one cause of death in children under the age of 15 years, affecting approximately 7,500 children each year (4). According to the Third National Cancer Survey for seven metropolitan areas and two states, representing roughly 10% of the United States population, the most common malignant tumors in children are: (a) leukemia; (b) tumors of the central nervous system; (c) tumors of the lymph tissue; (d) neuroblastoma; (e) Wilms' tumor; (f) osteosarcoma; (g) rhabdomyosarcoma; and (h) retinoblastoma (4). The primary difference between the adult and the pediatric patient is that the types of tumor most often affecting children are leukemia, embryonal tumors, and sarcomas, whereas adenocarcinomas and carcinomas are most frequently seen in adults (6).

Due to advances in research and technology, the child with cancer has a much better prognosis than a few years ago. The cure rate in the Pediatric Department at M. D. Anderson Hospital and Tumor Institute is 50%; that is, half of the children with cancer will stay in continuous or complete remission for an indefinite period of time without continued therapy (8). The overall goal of the health care team is to create an environment in which "normal" growth and development can be continued during the child's course of treatment.

131

COMMON MANIFESTATIONS

There are a number of factors that hinder normal growth and development. The patient may experience anorexia, nausea, vomiting, and diarrhea due to chemotherapy or radiotherapy, all of which will ultimately result in inadequate intake or inadequate utilization of nutrients. Other contributing factors that deter the efforts of the dietitian include increased metabolic requirements, psychological adjustment to the disease and hospitalization, family anxiety, and disruption of mealtime during the course of hospitalization.

Most children present with weight loss and a decreased appetite. Psychological adjustment, the illness itself, and debilitating treatment often cause an additional weight loss.

Anorexia significantly affects about 15% of cancer patients at the time of recurrence or spread of their cancers. Another 25% complain of early satiety, and, as the disease progresses, the degree of anorexia increases (7).

It is not uncommon for the child's caloric intake in the hospital to range from 0 to 800 kcal with a marked decrease in protein consumption. As the child responds to treatment, we generally see an increased caloric intake. However, one must remember that the course of treatment is usually several years and there is a continuous fluctuation in caloric intake. This fluctuation seldom allows for a constant or rapid weight gain. Also, cancer cells do not utilize energy as efficiently as normal cells. The protein-calorie deficient child has lessened resistance to therapy, and if malnutrition becomes chronic, there is a loss of immunity and the disease process may become irreversible (9). Therefore, good nutrition is essential in the treatment of the child with cancer.

NUTRITIONAL SUPPORT

Parent anxiety is a big factor to be considered in working with the pediatric patient. The family needs a tremendous amount of reinforcement and consolation. The family must be aware that the child will experience a decreased appetite, and it is not uncommon to see a significant weight loss. Many mothers become very upset when a child does not eat. To them, this is an obvious sign of the child's illness. In many homes as well as in the hospital, a child's eating habits and mealtime behavior sometimes create stress in both parent and child. Mealtime should be a relaxed atmosphere, and what the child eats is just as important as how much. Parents should be instructed in how to react to the child, e.g., instructing parents not to force foods when the child in experiencing nausea and vomiting.

During periods of extreme nausea, the patient may receive an antiemetic drug such as chlorpromazine, chlorohydrate, or prochlorperazine. According to recent studies at Washington University, food aversion is a learned behavior (1). Therefore, at M. D. Anderson Hospital favorite foods are discouraged during

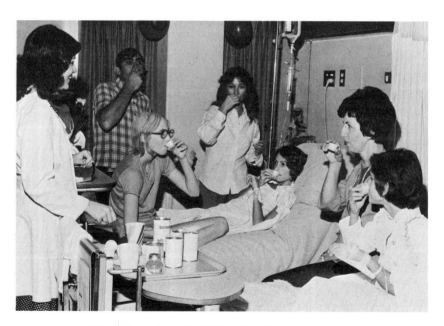

FIG. 1. Parents and children tasting supplements.

treatment, whereas juices, popsicles, and other nonaromatic cold foods are encouraged. It is during the period between treatments that one must be aggressive in nutritional build-up. Parents are instructed in methods of increasing calories as well as protein in the diet.

Supplements are used extensively at M. D. Anderson Hospital, and mothers are encouraged to take part in their preparation. Taste panels are conducted to discuss product availability and mixing procedures (Fig. 1). Some of the favorite supplements are milkshake-type drinks and eggnog. The best-tolerated nonmilk products are an orange flavored powdered supplement mixed with orange sherbet, and corn syrup solids mixed with juices.

Participation of the child in his own nutritional care plan is usually beneficial in achieving results; however, this is not always practical when the child is receiving debilitating therapies.

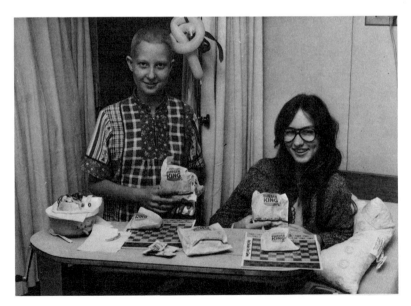

FIG. 2. Hamburger picnic is a special treat for the hospitalized patient.

The teenager who is feeling well tends to consume more calories if he keeps daily calorie counts and if one gives continuous feedback on results. This, however, is not true with the young child. Food games seem to create more interest, thus yielding better nutritional response with the young child.

Nutritious snacking is encouraged. Each week the volunteers sponsor a party with entertainment and refreshments. High protein foods such as pizza, Rice Krispie peanut butter bars, and punches with a milk base are encouraged, and we also serve the standard cake, cookies, and punch. The children receive nighttime snacks consisting of milkshakes, cheese and crackers, peanut butter crackers, and a variety of other foods. Also, once a week the children have a hamburger picnic sponsored by a local fast-food chain (Fig. 2).

The "mother's kitchen" located in the M. D. Anderson Hospital unit is a great asset in providing nutritional care for the pediatric patient. This is a small room with all facilities for food preparation. It is complete with refrigerator, burners, blender, microwave oven, and storage bins. Coffee is also available to parents. Staple foods are supplied by the Department of Dietetic Services, and the family brings any additional food they might want. This facility allows for participation of the family mem-

TABLE 1. *Utilization of kitchen by parents*[a]

Utilization	Percent using kitchen
Preparation of food for children	52
Daily	31
Three times per week	21
Storage of perishable or nonperishable food items for child only	27
Personal use only (coffee, etc.)[b]	21

[a] From ref. 8, with permission.
[b] This includes short stays in hospital or patients who cannot receive food postoperatively.

bers in the care of their child. It meets ethnic and religious needs that the hospital cannot provide. Most importantly, it gives the child an opportunity to have familiar foods at any time, day or night. Table 1 illustrates utilization of the kitchen (8).

NUTRITIONAL ASSESSMENT

A history of diet and typical food intake are taken to determine usual eating patterns, approximate caloric intake, and the nutritional status of the pediatric patient. A food array will help determine food preferences and variety in the diet. The child's status is plotted on a height-weight chart from the National Center for Health Statistics (2). The height-weight ratio allows for ethnic differences and seems to be more reliable than either height or weight used independently. Generally, anyone falling below the 10th percentile is considered malnourished; however, at this institution the 20th percentile is considered malnourished.

In working with amputees, one may use burn charts to determine body surface area. "The rule of nines" is one method of determining surface area percentages: head, arm, one quarter of the trunk or one half of a leg each equals 9% of the body surface. Infants and small children more exactly fit the "rule of sixes" because of larger heads and trunks and smaller extremities. The rule for infants is an arm, half of the head or leg and one eighth of the trunk each equals 6% of the body surface (3). Anthropometric measurements, which consist of arm circumference and triceps skinfold, may be used. In addition, one may obtain a subscapular skinfold or chest circumference; head circumference is used from birth to 36 months.

Biochemical values consisting of serum albumin, total iron binding capacity, creatinine/height index, nitrogen balance, and vitamin assays may be monitored. One must remember that, due to therapy as well as unique characteristics of the various types of tumors, certain biochemical values may not be true indicators of nutritional deficiency. For example, renal impairment caused by many chemotherapeutic drugs will result in an inaccurate creatinine/height index; serum vitamin B_{12} is decreased with leukemia; serum copper is increased with Hodgkins disease; and many children routinely have low hematocrit and low lymphocyte counts.

At M. D. Anderson Hospital, we routinely define overt malnourished children as those with: (a) low albumin according to age; (b) a height-weight ratio below the 20th percentile; and (c) poor nutritional intake over an extended period of time. Skin testing is not routinely used as a parameter in assessing the nutritional status of pediatric patients because children have not completely developed their immune response. The assessment used at this institution has been established to meet our specific needs, and is not an extensive evaluation, as used in research. By using a simple evaluation, more patients can be assessed and there are no additional fees to the patient.

HYPERALIMENTATION

When all means of oral nutritional support fail, intravenous hyperalimentation (IVH) may be indicated. IVH provides approximately 940 calories per liter using commercially available 50% dextrose and 8.5% amino acids (Table 2). Electrolytes. insulin, albumin, etc., may be added according to the patient's needs (5). Intra-lipid is administered once per week at 30 cc/kg up to 500 cc to prevent a fatty acid deficiency. This 10% fat emulsion is derived from soybean triglyceride and provides 1.1 calories/cc. Because it is an isotonic solution, it is suited for a peripheral vein.

A preliminary report of 20 children by Souchon et al. (5) indicates that the average intake of IVH was 1,800 calories/day for an average of 23.4 days and an average weight gain of 5 pounds. There was a low catheter-related sepsis rate with no complications due to catheter insertion. Therefore, with the safe

TABLE 2. *Intravenous hyperalimentation composition*[a]

Component	Amount per liter (total contents)	
Bottle IA		
Freamine II 8.5%	38.25 g	(3.8% of total)
Dextrose	225 g	(22.5% of total)
Sodium (as Freamine II and chloride)	44.5	meq
Potassium (as phosphate and chloride)	24.4	meq
Calcium (as gluconate)	500	mg
Phosphorus (as Freamine II and phosphate)	232.5	mg
Magnesium (as sulfate)	10	meq
Zinc (as sulfate)[b]	1.0	mg
Copper (as sulfate)[b]	0.5	mg
Fluoride (as sodium salt)[b]	25	μg
Iodide (as sodium salt)[b]	147.5	μg
Manganese (as sulfate)[b]	0.5	mg
MVI concentrate	2.0	ml
Vitamin K	1.0	mg
Folic Acid	1.0	mg
Vitamin B$_{12}$	10	μg
Bottle IB		
Freamine II 8.5%	38.25 g	(3.8% of total)
Dextrose 50%	225 g	(22.5% of total)
Sodium (as Freamine II and chloride)	44.5	meq
Potassium (as phosphate and chloride)	24.4	meq
Phosphorus (as Freamine II and phosphate)	232.5	meq

[a] From ref. 5, with permission.
[b] Contained in 2.5 ml of trace element solution.

and effective use of hyperalimentation, malnutrition is no longer an immediate threat to the pediatric cancer patient.

CONCLUSION

The pediatric cancer patient requires special nutritional care during his course of treatment. Therefore, the dietitian must continually be aware of the child's needs and give individual support. It is equally important for the entire health care team to strive for optimal nutrition so these children will grow and develop normally.

REFERENCES

1. Bernstein, I. L., Wallace, M. J., Bernstein, I. D., Bleyer, W. A., Chard, R. L., and Hartman, J. R. (1978): Learned food aversions in children receiving chemotherapy. *Science,* 200:1302–1303.
2. National Center for Health Statistics (1976): NCHS Growth Charts. Monthly Vital Statistics Report 25, No. 3, Suppl. (HRA) 76–1120. Health Resources Administration, Rockville, Maryland.
3. Nelson, W., Vaughan, V., and McKay, J. (1969): *Textbook of Pediatrics,* p. 230. W. B. Saunders Co., Philadelphia.
4. Safyer, A., and Miller, R. (1977): Childhood cancer; etiologic clues from epidemiology. *J. Sch. Health,* 47 (13):158–164.
5. Souchon, E., Cohen, B., Copeland, E., van Eys, J., and Dudrick, S. (1978): Hyperalimentation in the pediatric oncology patient; preliminary report. (*in press*).
6. Sutow, W., Viette, T., and Fernbach, D., editors (1977): *Clinical Pediatric Oncology.* C. V. Mosby, St. Louis.
7. Theologides, A. (1977): Nutritional management of the patient with advanced cancer. *Postgrad. Med.,* 61:97–101.
8. van Eys, J. (1977): Nutritional therapy in children with cancer. *Cancer Res.* 37:2457–2461.
9. van Eys, J. (1978): Nutrition and cancer in children. *Cancer Bull.,* 30:93–97.

Nutritional Management of the Cancer Patient, edited by J. Wollard.
Raven Press, New York © 1979.

Enteral and Parenteral Elemental Nutrition

Joy Wollard

Department of Nutrition and Food Service, The University of Texas System Cancer Center M. D. Anderson Hospital and Tumor Institute, Houston, Texas 77030

Elemental diet is a name coined for diets utilizing the ultimate constituents of nutrients that are absorbed into the body. These diets utilize synthetic amino acids, protein hydrolysates, predigested protein, or a combination of these types. Although the term chemically defined diet refers specifically to those diets containing only synthetic amino acids as the source of protein, the better choice of terminology when referring to the group is defined formula diet. To simplify the terminology in this chapter, the diets will be referred to as *elemental, enteral,* and *parenteral.*

Elemental diets may contain, in addition to the protein or amino acids, various types of carbohydrates, fats, vitamins, and minerals in balanced physiological ratios. Commercial formulations are available for enteral nutrition, utilizing the gastrointestinal (GI) tract, or parenteral nutrition, utilizing the venous system in a central vein for complete nutritional support. Peripheral appendage administration of total nutrition may be employed for short periods with a lesser dilution of solution than employed when using the central venous vessels. Figures 1 and 2 illustrate these modes of receiving nutrition.

This chapter will be devoted to the characteristics of elemental diets, their indications for use, commercial formulations, relative costs, modes of administration, complications and limitations, and, most important for the dietetic profession, the role of the dietitian in elemental nutrition.

141

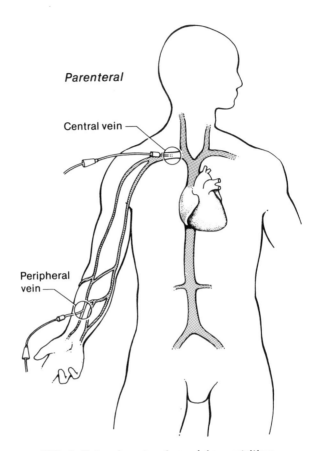

FIG. 1. Enteral route of receiving nutrition.

ENTERAL ELEMENTAL NUTRITION

Enteral elemental nutrition has characteristics that include:

1. Clear liquid
2. Relatively bulk free, producing one stool in 7 to 8 days (10)
3. Low in fat
4. Contains no lactose
5. Requires minimal digestion
6. Minimizes gastric, biliary, and pancreatic secretions

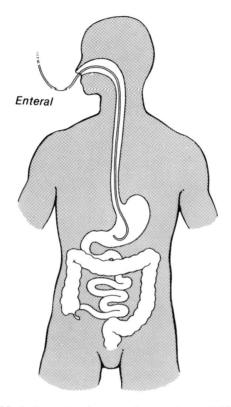

Enteral

FIG. 2. Parenteral route of receiving nutrition.

7. Reduces intestinal flora
8. Nonallergenic
9. Has approximately 500 to 850 mOsm/kg
10. Has the nutrient components of the diet absorbed in the proximal end of the intestine
11. Has a bitter flavor

The synthetic amino acids and protein hydrolysates used in the formulation characteristically have a bitter flavor that somewhat limits oral ingestion. Although this can be compounded in the cancer patient who frequently has an altered taste acuity, it can also be an advantage in that the taste may not be perceived as being bitter. The dietitian can aid patient acceptance of the product by suggesting various flavors the patient might find acceptable or by having the product made into gelatins, slushes, or frozen as a popsicle. The gelatin seems most successful in masking bitterness.

We find many studies that give insight into the formulations of the elemental diets that will be helpful in making product selections. Keep in mind that studies are frequently made of small isolated groups and findings may vary. Silk's studies indicate that a combination of protein hydrolysates with certain amino acids increases the efficiency of utilization, over free amino acids alone (8). Casein or collagen hydrolysates may be preferable as protein sources. Voitk states that the pancreas is stimulated by proteins and peptones, but not by pure amino acids. In the event of a diseased pancreas, one might want to consider limiting products containing peptide linkages (12). The importance of having knowledge of various studies is helpful in working with cancer patients because of their variable dysfunctional processes of digestion and absorption.

The rule of thumb in selecting the mode of nutritional intake is to use the GI tract if it is functional and if there are no complications, such as extreme nausea and vomiting. The only other contraindication for using a functional GI tract is when a condition such as anorexia exists that limits the caloric intake necessary to meet the metabolic needs of the patient. Although low stool production is seen with elemental nutrition, a patient should have bowel sounds without evidences of obstruction when using the diet. There have been instances of utilizing elemental nutrition without bowel sounds, but this frequently adds complications.

INDICATIONS FOR ENTERAL ELEMENTAL NUTRITION

Table 1 illustrates the indications for using enteral elemental nutrition as well as general causes of the conditions and the beneficial effects of the diet.

TABLE 1. *Indications for using enteral elemental nutrition*

Area of involvement[a]	Cause	Beneficial effect of elemental nutrition
GI tract lesions	Tumor or treatment	Hastens healing; decreases discomfort
Inflammatory GI tract regional enteritis iletitis	Chemotherapy or radiation therapy	Hastens healing; decreases discomfort
Short bowel syndrome	Massive resections	Lessens diarrhea secondary to overtaxed gut and aggravated by digestive juices
Malabsorption	Tumor or treatment	Assures proper ratio of ultimate constituents of nutrients presented
Acute pancreatitis		Allows the gland to rest by not being stimulated
Fistulas	Tumor or treatment	Hastens healing
Malnourished or depleted patient	Tumor or treatment	Aids nutritional build-up
Preoperative bowel preparation		Facilitates low stool production
Weaning from IVH or to supplement IVH		Gives additional nutrition and utilizes the GI tract, making it functional

[a] From ref. 4, with permission.

PRODUCT SELECTION

Because of the wide range of tumor influence upon digestion, absorption, and utilization of nutrients, it is imperative that dietitians have a good working knowledge of the characteristics of various diets. Having the ability to suggest the proper diet for a specific problem not only helps the patient but enhances the position of the dietitian on the health care team.

In selecting a commercial product or combination of products for a patient, criteria should include achieving a calorie/nitrogen ratio of 150 calories per gram of nitrogen for protein sparing (1), and having 4% of the caloric intake supplied from essential fatty acids, to prevent essential fatty acid (EFA) deficiency (5). There are many products available, some with a broad usage and some meeting specific dietary needs. Table 2 shows specific product information. These products range in cost from about 15 to 30 dollars per day.

TUBE PLACEMENT AND ADMINISTRATION
OF DIET

If the patient is to be tube fed, the tube selection and placement are extremely important (6). These topics will be discussed in the chapter on tube feedings. It has been found that elemental diets by tube are tolerated in higher concentrations when the tube is placed in the stomach rather than in the small bowel (C. P. Page et al., *unpublished paper*). Patients such as head and neck cancer patients, with limitations of intake confined to mechanical problems, tolerate intermittent hypertonic bolus feedings. In other patients this feeding method may cause abdominal cramping, diarrhea, nausea, and vomiting. Therefore, an alternative method of administering the elemental diet may need to be employed.

A continuous gavage drip is frequently the most successful method, beginning with a half-strength solution and increasing the density after 24 hr if the patient is free from complications and adverse side effects. The concentration should be advanced gradually, but progressively. Should complications arise at any time, the concentration should be dropped back to the last well-tolerated level. The initial rate of administration should be about 50 ml/hr. The patient should be observed for gastric distention, diarrhea, or glucosuria and advanced as tolerated, until the desired level is achieved. Within 3 days, the level could be up to 3 liters per day, if needed. Hyperosmolar solutions can be utilized, but should be used with care to avoid complications (9).

COMPLICATIONS OF ENTERAL ELEMENTAL NUTRITION

The complications from enteral elemental nutrition are generally obvious from the onset and relatively easy to manage (4). Simply dropping back to the last tolerated concentration and administration level will resolve any adverse side effects, as these side effects are caused from giving the patient too much diet too fast. The patient should be carefully observed from initiation of the enteral elemental diet for the following two frequently observed adverse side effects:

1. Hyperglycemia: Caused by osmotic diuresis secondary to glycosuria. When this occurs urine sugar and acetone should be checked at least every 6 hr and daily blood sugar counts taken until the situation stabilizes. Routine electrolytes, BUN, and liver function tests should be monitored. Potassium levels also need to be monitored.

2. Dumping and diarrhea: Caused by excessive volumes of hyperosmolar solutions going into the stomach and small intestines.

PARENTERAL ELEMENTAL NUTRITION

The search for a substitute for oral nutrition began over 300 years ago with Sir Christopher Wren (11). Carbohydrates in

TABLE 2. Composition of commonly used defined formula diets (per 1,000 kcal)[a]

Name of product	Grams protein and source	Grams fat and source	Grams CHO and source	Grams N_2/liter[b]	Volume to give 1,000 calories	Volume needed to meet 100% RDA	Water (Osm/kg)
Flexical	22.4 Amino acids and hydrolyzed casein	34.0 27.4–Soy oil 6.6–MCT oil	154.0 100.9–Sugar 48.4–Dextrin 4.7–Citrate	3.5	1,000	2,000	723
Precision, H.N.	41.7 Egg white solids	0.5 Vegetable oil Monodiglycerides	206.7 193.9–Malto-dextrin 12.8–Sugar	7.0	950	2,950	557
Precision, Isotonic	30.0 Egg white solids	31.3 Vegetable oil Monodiglycerides	150.0 Malto-dextrin and sugar	4.6	1,042	1,560	300
Precision, LR	23.7 Egg white solids	0.7 Vegetable oil Monodiglycerides	224.7 209.4–Malto-dextrin 15.3–Sugar	4.2	900	1,710	500–545
Precision, Mod. N.	32.5 Egg white solids	31.0 Vegetable oil Monodiglycerides	150.0 114.2–Malto-dextrin 35.8–Sugar	6.34	825	1,650	395

Vital	41.25	Amino acids and hydrolyzed proteins (soy, wheat, and meat)	10.23	Sunflower oil	183.15	Glucose oligosaccharides and polysaccharides; Sucrose, cornstarch	7.06	1,000	1,500	450
Vivonex	20.4	Crystalline amino acids	1.4	Safflower oil	226.3	Glucose oligosaccharides	3.26	1,000	1,800	Unflavored 500
Vivonex, H.N.	45.6	Crystalline amino acids	0.9	Safflower oil	202.4	Glucose oligosaccharides	7.29	1,000	3,000	850

[a] From ref. 8, with permission, and manufacturer's literature.
[b] When mixed according to manufacturer's directions.

limited amounts have been tolerated by humans in intravenous preparations since that time, but this does not allow the process of tissue growth and repair to be ongoing. It was not until the 1940s that scientists learned to incorporate protein as amino acids into i.v. solutions. In the early 1960s, Swedish investigators found a successful formula to increase i.v. calories utilizing soybean oil fractions and egg yolk phospholipids as emulsifiers.

It was not until S. J. Dudrick's investigation with dogs, also in the early 1960s, that a formula and mode of administration was established to allow successful parenteral elemental diet called intravenous hyperalimentation (IVH) or total parenteral nutrition (TPN) to be used (3). In his studies, Dr. Dudrick found he could induce total nutrition to meet hypermetabolic needs into the superior vena cava (Fig. 2), which would allow rapid dissemination of a hypertonic solution that would be tolerated.

The most important factor involved in the use of IVH in the cancer patient is to provide a caloric level to meet the demands of hypermetabolic states that prevent body wasting while at the same time providing a proper ratio of amino acids and other nutrients for growth and/or repair to tissue. Studies by Dr. Murray Copeland summarize the benefits received by the cancer patient when using IVH as an adjunctive treatment (2).

PATIENT SELECTION FOR IVH

Patients who are good candidates to receive IVH may be divided into the following categories:

1. Those having gastrointestinal disorders—much the same as in enteral elemental nutrition with the addition of:
    A. Extreme nausea: Caloric levels cannot be maintained. This is frequently seen in the cancer patient.
    B. Obstructions: IVH maintains good nutrition while allowing the bowel to rest, decreases the volume of up-

per gastrointestinal secretions, in addition to promoting healing by allowing a positive nitrogen balance and excess calories. IVH does not require a functioning bowel, as the GI tract is bypassed.

2. Patients in hypermetabolic states
   A. Burns
   B. Major trauma to the body or tissue: These patients undergo massive tissue breakdown and require a larger amount of calories and protein to rebuild body tissue and stores than can be ingested by oral nutrition. IVH is often used as adjunctive nutrition in the cancer patient, particularly in chemotherapy or radiotherapy when the patient is unable or unwilling to eat enough.

IVH COMPOSITION

The major proportions of calories in IVH are provided from dextrose, fructose, or invert sugars and act in the role of protein sparing for the amino acids to be utilized as a source of nitrogen rather than energy. Usually 2,000 to 3,000 calories of commercial IVH preparations will be sufficient to maintain nitrogen balance and prevent catabolism.

Each liter of IVH contains 250 g of glucose, which necessitates adequate pancreatic output of insulin or the careful addition of insulin to the solution. Parenteral hyperalimentation, like enteral, is gradually built up in dosage and equal care is taken in tapering off to prevent a hypoglycemic state. Enteral elemental nutrition is frequently utilized in this tapering off period, in addition to the IVH.

Many commercial formulas are available and can be somewhat modified by adjusting the electrolytes, trace elements, and vitamins. Table 3 illustrates the components of the seven commercially prepared IVH products most commonly used at M. D. Anderson Hospital. These products, with vitamins and electrolytes added, have a patient cost of about 35 dollars per liter, with the normal intake being about 3 liters per day. When a

TABLE 3. Composition of diluted, commonly used IVH preparations[a]

	Aminosol 5% (700 ml)	Travasol (8.5%) with electrolytes (500 ml)	Travasol (8.5%) without electrolytes (500 ml)	Aminosyn (7%) (500 ml)	Aminosyn (10%) (500 ml)	Freamine II (8.5%) (500 ml)	Nephramine (250 ml)
Protein source	Fibrin	Soybean	Soybean	Soybean	Soybean	Soybean	Soybean
Gram utilizable nitrogen	3.9	7.15	7.15	5.5	7.86	6.25	1.5
Calorie/nitrogen ratio (final dilution)	194:1	119:1	119:1	155:1	108:1	136:1	815:1
Essential amino acids (mg/100 ml)							
Leucine	636	526	526	660	940	770	880
Phenylalanine	100	526	526	310	440	480	880
Methionine	100	492	492	280	400	450	880
Lysine	400	492	492	510	720	620	640
Isoleucine	218	406	406	510	720	590	560
Valine	163	390	390	560	800	560	650
Threonine	232	356	356	370	520	340	400
Tryptophan	50	152	152	120	166	130	200
Semi-essential amino acids (mg/100 ml)							
Histidine	116	372	372	210	300	240	—
Arginine	290	880	880	690	980	310	—
Electrolytes (meq in final dilution)							
Na	7	35	—	—	—	5	1.5
K	1.2	30	—	2.7	2.7	—	—
Ca	—	—	—	—	—	—	—
Mg	—	5	—	—	—	—	—
Cl	—	35	17	—	—	—	—
HPO$_4$ (phosphate)	—	30	—	—	—	10	—
Acetate	—	65	26	—	—	—	—

[a] Bill Dana, Ph.D., M. D. Anderson Hospital Drug Information Services, *personal communication.*

patient exhibits a low albumin level or when stores need to be rapidly increased, albumin may be added to the solution at a cost of about 58 dollars for 12.5 g. As much as 25 g per bottle is added, which can make the total cost 140 dollars per liter or 420 dollars per patient day, if added to all three bottles. One addition of 25 g should be adequate to reverse the undesirable albumin level. The albumin has the added effect of preventing insulin losses from the container, in the event insulin is added to the solution.

COMPLICATIONS FROM IVH

There are many complications from IVH. The major ones that would cause the greatest contraindications are infection and contamination at the entrance site, cardiovascular overload, and glycosuria and hyperglycemia seen in enteral elemental nutrition. Prolonged use of IVH for a period of more than 3 months can cause a fatty acid deficiency that is evidenced by skin lesions. This can be avoided with the administration of a peripheral IV product such as Intralipid, which is a 10% fat emulsion and costs the patient about 35 dollars for a 500 cc bottle. This is also a source of additional calories. EFA deficiency can also be reversed by rubbing safflower oil on the skin.

ADVANTAGES OF IVH AND COMPARISON TO ENTERAL ELEMENTAL NUTRITION

The main advantages of using IVH over enteral nutrition are that it can be used when nausea is present and without a functioning gut. IVH has the capability of a more rapid nutritional build-up than enteral nutrition. The advantages of the enteral mode of nutrition are the greater safety found from a less invasive technique of administration, a greater leeway in providing vitamins and micronutrients, the fact that fats can easily and safely be administered with the solution, and that enteral nutrition is by far the less expensive mode of receiving elemental nutrition.

THE ROLE OF THE DIETITIAN IN ELEMENTAL NUTRITION

The role of the clinical dietitian in elemental nutrition is extremely important to the health care team. Being trained to help make nutritional assessments and evaluations aids in the decision process of the type and content of nutrition needed by the patient. Dietitians are trained to monitor and recommend trace elements, vitamins, and electrolytes that should be added or modified. The dietitian also helps monitor the fatty acid status of the patient. From the dietary history, valuable information is afforded the health care team. Recognizing dietitians' expertise in the field of nutrition, patients will accept encouragement and assistance with nutrition education. This should assure maintenance of optimal nutrition and shorten the period needed to wean a patient from elemental nutrition back to conventional nutritional practices.

REFERENCES

1. Blackburn, G. L., and Bristrian, B. (1977): Nutritional support resources in hospital practice. In: *Nutritional Support of Medical Practice,* edited by H. Schneider, C. E. Anderson, and D. B. Coursins, pp. 139–151. Harper and Row Publishers, Hagerstown, Maryland.
2. Copeland, E. M., and Dudrick, S. J. (1976): Intravenous hyperalimentation as adjunctive treatment. In: *The Cancer Patient.* Clinical Digest, 6:1–4.
3. Dudrick, S. J., Willmore, D. W., Vars, H. M., and Rhodes, J. E. (1968): Long-term total parenteral nutrition with growth, development, and positive nitrogen balance. *Surgery,* 64:134–142.
4. Kaminski, M. V., Jr. (1976): Enteral hyperalimentation. *Surg. Gynecol. Obstet.,* 143:12–16.
5. Kark, R. M. (1974): Liquid formula and chemically defined diets. *J. Am. Diet Assoc.,* 64:476–479.
6. Page, C. P., Ryan, J. A., and Haff, R. C. (1976): Continual

catheter administration of an elemental diet. *Surg. Gynecol. Obstet.*, 142:184–188.

7. Shils, M., Bloch, A., and Chernoff, R. (1976): Liquid formulas for oral and tube feeding. *Clin. Bull.*, 6:151.
8. Silk, D. B. A., Marrs, T. C., Addison, J., Burston, D., Clark, M. L., and Matthews, D. M. (1973): Absorption of amino acids from an amino acid mixture stimulating casein and a tryptic hydrolysate of casein in man. *Clin. Sci. Mol. Med.*, 45:715–719.
9. Winborn, A. L., Kaminski, M. V., Jr., Hoppe, M. L., and Aquinas, M. (1977): Hyperosmolar feeding solutions with the avoidance of diarrhea. *JPEN*, 1:4.
10. Winitz, M., Stedman, D. A., and Graff, J. (1970): Studies in metabolic nutrition employing chemically defined diets—I and II. *Am. J. Clin. Nutr.*, 23:525.
11. Dudrick, S. J., and Roads, J. E. (1971): New horizons for intravenous feedings. *JAMA*, 215:939–949.
12. Voitk, A., Brown, R. A., Echave, V., McArole, A. H., Gurd, F. N., and Thompson, A. G. (1973): Use of an elemental diet in the treatment of complicated pancreatitis. *Am. J. Surg.*, 125:223–227.

Nutritional Management of the Cancer Patient, edited by J. Wollard.
Raven Press, New York © 1979.

Tube Feeding and the Head and Neck Cancer Patient

Kathleen Bradford

Department of Nutrition and Food Service, The University of Texas System Cancer Center M. D. Anderson Hospital and Tumor Institute, Houston, Texas 77030

The health care team gives high priority to the nutritional care of the tube fed patients and the dietitian plays an important role in assessing the needs of these patients. She recommends formulations and encourages patients to accept an unorthodox and often socially repugnant means of receiving nutrition.

When mechanical impediments to chewing or swallowing exist and the intestinal tract is functional, feeding tubes can provide the means for a nutritionally complete and balanced diet. Impairments that might render an individual dependent upon tube feedings include radical surgery or obstructing tumors in the oral cavity, esophagus, or stomach, as well as neurological problems and mental disturbances. Severe stomatitis resulting from chemotherapy and radiation can decrease the intake of liquids and solid foods, thus necessitating tube feedings as a total replacement diet or a supplementary means of intake. In the majority of these cases, when biting, chewing, and swallowing become painful experiences, feeding by tube can ensure adequate nutritional intake. Tube feedings are also indicated with many prolonged problems of digestion as well as in anorexia, when a patient will not or cannot eat enough.

At M. D. Anderson Hospital, the majority of the feeding tubes are used with head and neck cancer patients. Many factors compound the nutritional toll of these patients. They are usually males over 50 years of age who have a history of cigarette smoking and heavy alcohol consumption. The result is manifested by a history of poor nutritional intake, frequently compounded by their being edentulous. A 15-pound to 20-pound weight loss is quite common in the initial presentation at the outpatient clinic. Obstructing tumors contribute significantly to this weight loss and treatment will further reduce the nutritional status.

PLACEMENT SITES

The different tube insertion sites made to accomodate enteral nutrition (Fig. 1) include: nasogastric, pharyngostomy,

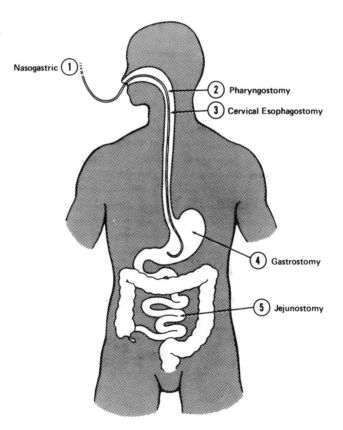

FIG. 1. Common placement for feeding tubes.

cervical esophagostomy, gastrostomy, and jejunostomy. Much surgery in the head and neck region results in a large amount of tissue loss or damage and, therefore, a reduction in body function requires temporary tube feedings for healing, or permanent tube feedings if adequate reconstruction cannot be made. Total laryngectomies, total or partial glossectomies, and mandible or maxillary resections are a few of the procedures requiring patients to be fed by nasogastric tube. Gastrostomies are used to bypass the head and neck area, while patients who have a jejunostomy tube will have their digestive systems bypassed.

TUBE SIZE

The length of tubes used for feedings ranges from about 15 to 20 inches, depending upon the insertion site. A nasogastric tube, for instance, that is too long will curl up in the patient's stomach and take up space needed for food, in addition to

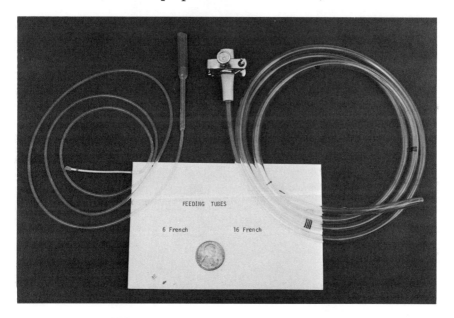

FIG. 2. Size comparison of feeding tubes.

being extremely uncomfortable for the patient. The diameter, measured in French sizes, varies from 5 to 18 inches; the larger the number, the wider the diameter. The size of the tubes is illustrated in Fig. 2 by comparison to a coin. Each size increases in increments of ⅓ mm. Commercially prepared liquid formulations can be administered through an 8F tube with little or no physical irritation to the patient (1); however, more viscous preparations will require larger tube diameters. Tube designs include one with a mercury-weighted tip, which aids in intubation and identification of placement (1). Tubing material is either polyvinyl or rubber, with polyvinyl being more widely used.

TUBE INSERTION

The patient's physician is responsible for inserting the tube. Tube insertion techniques are taught to nurses for care of hospitalized patients, while many patients using tubes in the home environment are encouraged to insert their own tubes. A slightly lubricated or chilled tube may be easier to insert; however, care must be exercised to avoid having a rigid tube as it may damage the alimentary canal. At M. D. Anderson Hospital, should platelet counts fall below 100,000 from therapy or disease, intubation is deferred due to the increased chance of bleeding. In these instances, hydration and alimentation are achieved through i.v.'s and oral feedings until the platelet counts increase.

LIQUID DIET FORMULATIONS

The array of commercial liquid diet formulations is extensive. (Please refer to the chapter on supplementation for a detailed description of types of products available for use.) The dietitian must have a thorough knowledge of the range of formulations from which to choose. These include nutritionally complete formulas of three types: (a) intact protein, milk-containing products; (b) intact protein, lactose-free; and (c) defined-formula diets. There are also many products and foods that can be adapted for supplemental use by the tube-feeding process.

Constant nutrients, sterilized formulations, and minimal preparation time are the advantages of commercially prepared formulas. Their disadvantage is that the formulations are fixed. As an alternate, pureed food formulas can be developed to meet the patient's needs. This ability to individualize the formula does not, in many instances, outweigh questionable sanitary preparation procedures and increased costs in both ingredients and labor (3).

ADMINISTRATION

Gravity drip or continuous infusion are the two methods by which formulas can be administered. Gravity drip is a method of administering bolus feeding utilizing a set-up as pictured in Fig. 3. This method can be administered successfully in the

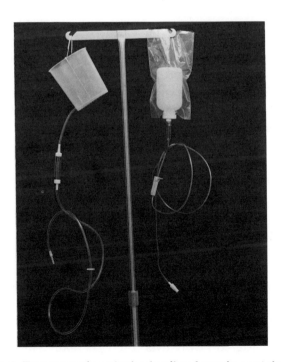

FIG. 3. Two examples of tube feeding formula containers.

home or the hospital. The bolus feeding is used primarily with patients who have limitations only in getting food into their stomachs.

GENERAL PROCEDURES FOR GRAVITY DRIP

The patient should be sitting upright during a feeding and remain in that position approximately an hour after the meal to avoid reflux or regurgitation. After 30 cc of water has been passed through the tube to ensure tube patency, the formula is introduced. The drip rate can be controlled by a screw clamp and by adjusting the height of the flask above the patient. The formula should be given slowly to minimize any distention, nausea, vomiting, cramps, or diarrhea. A continuous flow is necessary to prevent air from being introduced into the stomach. Length of a feeding can vary from 30 min to 1 hr; however, this is determined by the patient's tolerance, ability to help himself, and the volume of formula. As a rule, room-temperature formula seems best tolerated. At the end of each feeding, another 30 cc of water is poured through the tube to prevent occluding by the formula. Finally, the tube is clamped until the next feeding.

Individualizing the diet is very important. Taste may not be a factor, but individual preferences must be taken into account. M. D. Anderson Hospital patients are encouraged to incorporate familiar foods to their tube diets when possible. There seems to be a psychological advantage when a patient can include identifiable foods such as juice or coffee with cream and sugar along with a tube feeding formula. This also gives the patient the opportunity to stir and smell foods such as coffee, to satisfy the other senses.

POSTSURGICAL PATIENTS UTILIZING GRAVITY DRIP

The postsurgical patient will best tolerate a gravity drip diet that is administered slowly over a long period. Within 24 to 48 hr after surgery, when proper bowel sounds are evident, the physician should order the tube diet to begin. The diet on the first day consists of clear liquids such as juice, coffee, and broth, to confirm the patient's tolerance to foods. Initially feedings of 300 to 500 cc are offered every 3 to 4 hr to establish tolerance. The second day, half-strength formula, usually a lactose-free product, is given followed by full-strength formula on the third day. On the fourth day, the diet progression and the volume of the feeding are adjusted to meet the patient's calorie requirements. If this progression is not readily tolerated, one must be designed to meet the patient's specific level of tolerance.

THE NONSURGICAL PATIENT UTILIZING GRAVITY DRIP

Generally, patients requiring tube feedings who have not had surgery are ones who cannot or will not eat enough to maintain a positive nitrogen balance and stabilized weight. Care must be taken after the tube has been inserted to ensure that the patient can tolerate the selected formulation and to establish the level of intake. Half-strength, lactose-free formulas may need to be used at intervals of every 3 to 4 hr. Patients can be built up to take as many as 3,000 calories or 3,000 cc daily if needed.

CONTINUOUS INFUSION

Continuous infusion ensures adequate nutritional intake with minimal adverse side-effects in patients who have decreased digestive and absorptive abilities. Continuous infusion apparatus, as illustrated in Fig. 3, is used to administer formula in a constant flow at a specified rate. It slowly introduces the formula throughout a 24-hr period to avoid fluctuations. This method frequently allows a greater amount of nutrition to be taken into the body since normal rest periods are utilized. With continuous infusion, half-strength feedings are begun at 50 cc per hour. Formula strength and rate of infusion increases to full-strength and as great as 125 cc per hour within a few days, according to the patient's tolerance. Tolerance levels can be built up to utilize hyperosmolar solutions, if indicated (4).

The formula for the day should be divided into six containers that should be changed every four hours to prevent bacteria growth or contamination. The tube should be irrigated with 30 cc of water to avoid occluding by the formula between each container.

The feeding can be given to the patient in any position; however, a disadvantage to continuous infusion is in having the patient confined throughout the duration of the feeding. As this could last from a few days to several weeks, continuous drip is better accepted by the patient who is bedridden than the patient who is ambulatory. This method of infusion is, therefore, seldom used in a home situation.

DIET PROGRESSION IN THE HEAD AND NECK CANCER PATIENT AFTER TUBE REMOVAL

The time factor involved in advancing the patient's diet to liquid and solid foods by mouth is highly proportional to the extent of surgery performed, the healing rate, the necessity for reconstruction, and the presence of the needed oral structures for swallowing. Once the physician has observed that the patient is able to swallow his own saliva, the patient is asked to swallow water to check for a fistula in the operative area. If healing appears to be "airtight," a diet by mouth is ordered.

The conclusion has been reached that deglutition is initially more successful with semisolid foods such as custard or very thin mashed potatoes, rather than clear liquids. Not all head and neck cancer patients are eating by mouth at the time of discharge, however. Many are discharged when able to take only liquids or pureed foods. More than likely, this diet is nutritionally incomplete; therefore, stressing supplementation and fortification of the diet is the major emphasis in discharge planning and dietary consultations. Since a large percentage of the patients being discharged enter radiotherapy programs, adequate nutrition is especially important.

FLUID INTAKE

Fluid intake should not be ignored while a patient is being tube fed. The average adult requires approximately 2,000 to 2,500 cc water per day (2). For the patient on tube feedings, the formula, incidental water intake, and additional beverages through the day provide well over the average need. Individual differences as well as fever, alter fluid requirements; hence, an adjustment may be necessary for some patients.

ORAL HYGIENE

Oral hygiene is of the utmost importance and must not be neglected while a patient is on tube feedings. Even though the mouth is not the primary route of nourishment, tooth brushing and oral irrigations should continue. This can contribute to the decrease of the bacteria count in the oral cavity and in turn decrease the likelihood of infections that could be detrimental, especially if the surgery was in the oral cavity.

ROLE OF THE DIETITIAN

The role of the dietitian is quite significant in the implementation of tube feedings. Most often the dietitian is the only member of the health care team who knows exactly which formulas are available to the patient. In determining the most adequate tube feeding formula for each patient, the following factors should be kept in mind: (a) dietary modification (lactose-free, low sodium, etc.); (b) tolerance; (c) osmolality; (d) acceptability; (e) convenience; (f) cost; and (g) availability of the formula to the patient at discharge. The dietitian is able to manipulate the available formulas to best suit the dietary needs of the patient.

To ensure maximum care of patients who have head and neck cancer, it is imperative that the lines of communication remain open between all members of the health care team and include conferences, documentation of pertinent facts, and continuing nutrition education.

REFERENCES

1. Dobbie, R. P., and Hoffmeister, J. A., (1976): Continuous pump-tube enteric hyperalimentation. *Surg. Gynecol. Obstet.,* 143:273–276.
2. Goodhart, R. S., and Shils, M. E., editors (1973): *Modern Nutrition in Health and Disease,* 5th edition, p. 410. Lea and Febiger, Philadelphia.
3. Horsh, D. J., (1966): A cost analysis of tube feeding procedures. *Hospitals,* 40:1–4.
4. Winborn, A. L., Kaminiski, M. V., Jr., Hoppe, M. C., and Aquinas, S. M., (1977): Hyperosmolar feeding solutions with avoidance of diarrhea. *JPEN,* 1:4.

Nutritional Management of the Cancer Patient, edited by J. Wollard.
Raven Press, New York © 1979.

Nutrition Rehabilitation: A Modality of Behavior Modification

Paula K. Hoffman

Department of Nutrition and Food Service, The University of Texas System Cancer Center M. D. Anderson Hospital and Tumor Institute, Houston, Texas 77030

Rehabilitation of the cancer patient is becoming an area of concern in oncology. The emphasis in any form of rehabilitation is on helping the patient adjust to his present state rather than allowing him to dwell on what he was in the past. Ironically, modern oncology places greater emphasis on destroying neoplastic cells with little attention given to the nutritional consequences of the treatment (7). Since the disease and its treatment have direct effects on the nutritional state of the patient, nutrition plays a major role in his rehabilitation.

Nutrition rehabilitation is the restoration of patients who have residual deficits as a consequence of their disease, or treatment to as normal a state of nutritional health as possible (16). It also involves teaching patients new eating habits and making them feel comfortable with their eating patterns while meeting their nutritional needs. Candidates for nutrition rehabilitation include those exhibiting obvious weight loss prior to treatment, during treatment, or upon return visits, and those given permanent or temporary modified diets.

PROBLEMS ENCOUNTERED IN REHABILITATION

The problems specific to rehabilitating cancer patients are weight loss, anorexia, adjustment to a new eating style, pain, and motivation. Since most patients continue receiving treatment during rehabilitation therapy, the problems associated with radiotherapy, chemotherapy, and surgery are pertinent here as well.

One of the most obvious complications in cancer patients is weight loss, which is constantly associated with anorexia. Although anorexia is described as an important cause of protein-calorie malnutrition, its mechanism is still poorly understood. While it may be related to therapy or disease, a transient anorexia, the result of emotional distress, can be defined (9). This distress can occur at initial diagnosis, at diagnosis of recurrent disease, or during periods of pain and discouragement. The observation of an aversity to food directly related to behavior supports relearning a positive nutritional pattern, but there is a need for a more definitive protocol for this type of anorexia.

Another problem associated with nutrition rehabilitation is adjustment to a new style of eating. This adjustment is not, as one might expect, so much a physical problem as a social problem. Taste stimulation from a juicy sirloin steak is no longer present when served in the ground meat or blenderized meat version. The food substances can be the same as served a regular diet with modification in consistency. However, often the sight and odors from the new food styles make the patient and those eating with him very self-conscious.

The reaction of the patient's family to the diet change plays an important part in the patient's reaction. For example, the wife who eats lunch with her husband in the dining room or at a bedside and responds, "How can you eat that way?" is repulsed at the thought of having to prepare food in such a manner when her husband returns home. Once removed from the hospital setting, the patient often encounters an even more discouraging problem. A society as structured as ours to fast food operations and eating out, allows little leeway for the person who needs modifications in food consistency. It's hard to find a McDonald's that will prepare a pureed Big Mac.

Pain, too, can be one of the most noted deterrents to rehabilitation. Pain increases the dependency and self-centeredness of the patient (13). The pain is real but out of control, to the extent that it monopolizes the patient's life. At M. D. Anderson Rehabilitation Center there are malnourished patients who are clinically diagnosed as having "no known evidence of disease." However, these patients describe a ferocious pain that forbids normal body functioning, including eating.

Often motivation is found to be the biggest enemy of all in nutrition rehabilitation. Motivation can be defined as the desire to interact successfully with one's environment (1), and is truly an intrinsic quality. Cancer patients are sometimes more comfortable in a sheltered situation such as the hospital or rehabilitation center, rather than at home. The lack of motivation in cancer patients is understandable, as many of them have physical deformities or prostheses, have lost their jobs, or are experiencing family problems, all directly related to the word "cancer." In rehabilitation, a combination of intensified support, education, and teamwork is necessary to encourage and build motivation.

BEHAVIOR MODIFICATION

According to MacDonald, general supportive measures tend to be more effective than drugs or hormone therapy in dealing with the difficult problems of anorexia, and sensory abnormalities of taste and smell associated with malignancy (11). The initial response to the need for nutritional support in the cancer patient is total parenteral nutrition (TPN). Although TPN is definitely useful in nutritional support, such intervention takes place long after the beginning of malnutrition is evident. Many patients would benefit from a concentrated enteral nutritional program at the beginning of the treatment stage.

Another supportive therapy technique is behavior modification in an effort to change the patient's eating behavior and attitude toward his diet. Behavior modification is the systematic application of basic learning techniques to change behavior toward more constructive channels. Behavior therapy is aimed at acquiring, strengthening, and maintaining a new behavior and eliminating maladaptive behavior. It is based on the assumption that human beings are essentially shaped and determined by their sociocultural environments. In simple terms, human behavior is learned behavior, which suggests that some of the cancer patient's aversion to food is learned and can be changed (5).

Researchers have provided evidence that behavior therapy is effective in treating obesity (14). Although often neglected, studies have shown that the underweight patient and anorexic patient too can benefit from such therapy, even in a hospital setting (3,8). The main question, then, is how can these techniques be suitably applied to cancer patients?

Research has been initiated at Midwest Research Institute in Kansas City, Missouri, to study the application of behavior modification techniques in the treatment of anorexia in cancer patients. At Washington University, a study is being conducted involving children's selection of food during several courses of chemotherapy (4). At M. D. Anderson Rehabilitation Center, behavior modification in a simplified form is the basis for the entire nutritional program.

M. D. ANDERSON REHABILITATION CENTER

At M. D. Anderson Rehabilitation Center, the goal of the behavior modification program, a joint effort between the dietary and nursing departments, is for the patient to maintain his weight. The patient is taught how to meet his increased nutritional needs and how to adapt high-calorie eating patterns for home usage.

The main criterion for participation in the program is a 10 pound or 10 to 15% weight loss. The patient is interviewed by the dietitian and instructed on high calorie meal supplementation. An individualized feeding schedule incorporating a variety of snacks is established with the patient.

A nutritional maintenance sheet, as illustrated in Fig. 1, is

FIG. 1. Nutritional maintenance worksheet is utilized as a motivational tool in behavior therapy.

FLOOR:_____

Nutritional maintenance worksheet

Room	Name	Suggested Supplement	WT	AM	PM	HS	T	WT	AM	PM	HS	T	WT	AM	PM	HS	T	WT	AM	PM	HS	T	WT	AM	PM	HS	T

used as a motivation mechanism of adherence to the program, and attached to the refrigerator door on each floor. The patient's name, daily weights, and supplements are listed, with a pencil attached to enable the patient to record his own feedings. Most patients adapt to such a schedule and become dependable to take their own supplement once weight gain or maintenance is realized.

The cafeteria-style dining room at M. D. Anderson Rehabilitation Center is a therapeutic modality in itself. All patients eat in the dining room including those fed per tube. The setting establishes a home-style atmosphere, as staff members and patients eat together. Many times a variety of conversations can be overheard, ranging from death and denial to daily jokes and laughter.

Adaptation to clientele is an important role of the food service at the rehabilitation center. At times, the center has an occupancy of 60% Mexican Americans. During these periods, the menu is adjusted to serve more Mexican entrees and typical Mexican items. In all matters, every effort is taken to make the meal time a pleasant one and as relaxed a situation as possible.

PROTOCOL FOR BEHAVIOR MODIFICATION

There are several basic steps to establishing a behavior modification protocol for patients (5, 15):

1. Observe and define the problem behavior.
2. Create a means of changing the behavior.
3. Educate the patient in ways to change the behavior.
4. Shape the behavior by stressing one small, achievable step at a time.
5. Measure the behavior and record feedback.
6. Evaluate the program.

The main therapeutic concern is to observe and define the problem behavior. In the cancer patient, this behavior is an inability to meet nutritional needs, usually exhibited by aversion to food or decreased food intake, as evidenced by weight loss. The primary problem may be anorexia, difficulty in swallowing, or taste abnormalities.

The second step is creating a means of changing such behavior. This step usually involves a series of smaller steps that should be attempted in sequence. For example, if Mr. B.'s problem is an inability to consume adequate calories in three meals to maintain his weight, steps toward a supplemental feeding program should be initiated by introducing one snack per day and gradually increasing this amount to six meals per day. Or, in the case of low protein intake, the progressive steps would be to discover protein foods well-tolerated and slowly incorporate them into the diet.

Education is an important tool in establishing and fulfilling these goals. The dietitian must be as creative as possible and encourage the patient to take an active role in the education process. Working together, the dietitian and patient determine a specific meal plan. The patient should be allowed to choose among several types of dietary supplemental plans, not only for variety but to give the patient a feeling of control. Additionally, the alert patient can keep a diary of daily food intake. The dietitian reviews the caloric needs of the patient and implements ways to meet these needs. A simple calorie counter is given to the patient to use in making food selections of high nutritional value. Records are kept in 24-hr periods and reviewed with the patient by the therapist. Such diaries have been successful in treating obesity but have not often been applied to the cancer patient. At M. D. Anderson Hospital Rehabilitation Center, such a technique was used with a 17-year-old sarcoma patient who had rapidly been losing weight. Not only were the diary and calorie counter at her side for every meal, but she was seen snacking enthusiastically on every free occasion.

Positive reinforcement should be utilized to encourage constructive changes in behavior (5), and the entire staff should be aware of weight gains and other accomplishments, and compliment the patient when he achieves his goals. Patient interaction also can be a positive reinforcement mechanism. Many times patients meet at the hospital, share experiences and beliefs regarding their diseases, and pass on helpful tips on how to deal with the complications of therapy.

The third step in establishing a behavior modification program is developing a means of measuring feedback and behavior. For the dietitian, the feedback that needs to be measured is weight versus caloric intake. Preferably, calorie counts should be conducted four times a week, including one weekend day. Other necessary information includes any changes in diagnosis, changes in patient's mood, and changes in treatment.

Evaluation of the program involves two areas. One is exploring what the patient is currently doing, i.e., weight versus intake, and comparing this action to prior patterns developed before his illness and subsequent treatment. The second phase is noting the percent of improvement derived from the program, taking into account staff time and cost.

VARIABLES IN BEHAVIOR THERAPY

The most influential variable in the behavior modification program is socialization among patients. If a patient is encouraged to eat with fellow patients or have guests come eat with him, a pleasurable experience can be made from what was a painful one.

Social interaction can encourage adaptation of new behavior. Although burdened with his own problems, the patient can always find others in similar situations to talk to. Often patients reach out to help other patients, thereby deriving comfort and a sense of purpose that lessens their own misery.

DIETITIAN'S ROLE

The cancer patient has been described as being "in limbo," a kind of "no man's land" where he does not know what the future will bring (12). Studies of the cancer patient have shown him to have three essential needs (10). The first is the need to maintain his own destiny, even if it is only the choice of what he eats for breakfast or the clothes he wears. He needs to be able to make decisions on his own. The second is that technical language and procedures, unfamiliar and frightening to most people, must be expressed in a form that he can understand. The third need of the cancer patient is an opportunity to share with someone his feelings of being unjustly robbed of life and full functioning.

The first way in which a dietitian can satisfy these needs is to be supportive. Support has been defined as simple conversation, a matter of professional competence involving the bedside manner (2). In conversation, the dietitian must be realistic and talk with the patient rather than take the role of an analyst. Today, support seems to have gone out of fashion, as hospital employees rush impersonally down halls, trying to accomplish as much as possible in each 24-hr day. Far too often the patients become room numbers rather than names, and general courtesy and thoughtfulness are forgotten.

A way with words is a dietitian's key advantage in support. In conversation, there is an important exchange of information with the patient and talk becomes an indispensable therapeutic tool. It relieves anxiety and increases comfort. Talk can also be a time-filler and time seems to be one thing the cancer patient has that moves too slowly (6).

Through small talk, a dietitian can discover problems that might have gone unnoticed. Attitudes conveyed to the patient by those who care for him directly affect how the patient feels about his diagnosis, and the dietitian must be honest, creative, and realistic in talking with the patient. The most potent weapon for successful rehabilitation is a positive attitude.

The second role of the dietitian in rehabilitation, and one most often accepted, is that of educator. The dietitian has a wealth of information that must be shared enthusiastically with the patient. Guidelines to good eating and suggestions for high calorie foods are extremely important for the cancer patient.

The dietitian must counter any false information the patient has received from other sources. Helpful hints dealing with therapy and anorexia are a means of educating the patient. Games based on nutrition or crossword puzzles of nutritional terms can be invented by the staff to increase patient interest.

Finally, the dietitian is a team member. A comprehensive, multidisciplinary, cooperative approach that involves all members of the health care team is currently emphasized in rehabilitation (13). The team at our rehabilitation center consists of a clinical psychologist, medical director, occupational therapist, physical therapist, chaplain, dietitians, nurses, and social service workers. The team's main objective is to meet the physical and psychological needs of the patient and to prepare him for resuming his home life. Once the patient's needs have been assessed, each department is made aware of its role in the patient's care. The team also enables the staff to more clearly understand the patient and his problems. By combining information about the patient's attitude from several departments, the staff is made aware of the patient's frustrations and his means of expressing them.

Another advantage of the team approach is the moral support it provides. Working with cancer patients can be very discouraging at times and an emotional experience for the staff member. At our rehabilitation center, a nonstructured means of support is in operation among team members. One feels free to discuss with others the anxieties and discouragements concerning certain patients. The members support each other in much the same way as they support the patients.

Rehabilitating the cancer patient, especially if his diagnosis is terminal, depends on the staff's sensitivity. The more conscious the staff is of the patient, the more likely he is to be invited back to life. The manner in which nutritional support is directed toward the patient can greatly effect his response to such information.

With longer survival rates in cancer patients, nutrition rehabilitation will have continual importance. The assurance of adequate nutritional education is the responsibility of the dietitian. However, the nutritional problems in cancer are both physical and social and require a team approach. Behavioral approaches in meeting nutritional goals offer a new means of nutritional support of the cancer patient.

REFERENCES

1. *American Heritage Dictionary,* edited by W. Morris. (1971): American Heritage Publishing Co. Inc., and Houghton Mifflin Co., Dallas.
2. Barclay, V. (1967): The crisis in cancer. *Am. J. Nurs.,* 67:278–280.
3. Blinder, B. J., Freeman, D., and Stunkard, A. J. (1970): Behavior therapy of anorexia nervosa: Effectiveness of activity as a reinforcer of weight gain. *Am. J. Psychiatry,* 126:1093–1098.
4. Berstein, I. L. (1978): Learned taste aversions in children receiving chemotherapy. *Science,* 200:1302–1303.
5. Corey, G. (1977): Behavior therapy. In: *Theory and Practice of Counseling and Psychotherapy,* pp. 117–141. Brooks/Cole Publishing Co., Monterey, California.
6. Crayton, J. (1969): Talking with persons who have cancer. *Am. J. Nurs.,* 69:744–748.
7. Donaldson, S. S. (1977): Nutritional consequences of radiotherapy. *Cancer Res.,* 37:2407–2413.
8. Gulanick, N., Woodburn, L. T., and Rinm, D. C. (1975): Weight gain through self-control procedures. *J. Consult. Clin. Psychol.,* 43:536–539.
9. Holland, J. C. B., Rowland, J., and Plummer, M. (1977): Psychological aspects of anorexia in cancer patients. *Cancer Res.,* 37:2428–2435.
10. Klagsburn, S. C. (1971): Communications in the treatment of cancer. *Am. J. Nurs.,* 71:944–948.
11. MacDonald, J. S., and Schein, P. S. (1976): Mechanism and management of malnutritional states in patients with cancer. *Clin. Gastroenterol.,* 5:809–816.
12. Shepardson, J. (1972): Team approach to the patient with cancer. *Am. J. Nurs.,* 72:488–491.
13. Smith, E. (1975): *A Comprehensive Approach to Rehabilitation of the Cancer Patient.* The University of Texas Health Science Center, Houston.
14. Stunkard, A. (1972): New therapies for the eating disorders. *Arch. Gen. Psychiat.,* 26:391–398.
15. Tullis, J. F., and Tullis, K. F. (1978): Obesity. In: *Nutritional*

Support of Medical Practice, edited by H. A. Schneider, C. E. Anderson, and D. B. Coursin, pp. 392–405. Harper and Row, Publishers, Hagerstown, Maryland.

16. U.S. Department of Health, Education and Welfare, National Institutes of Health/National Cancer Institute (1977): Cancer Program Objective 7.

Nutritional Management of the Cancer Patient, edited by J. Wollard.
Raven Press, New York © 1979.

Nutritional Supplementation

Debra E. Selig

Department of Nutrition and Food Service, The University of Texas System Cancer Center M. D. Anderson Hospital and Tumor Institute, Houston, Texas 77030

Supplementation is defined as the act of making complete, filling up, or making an addition. Therefore, nutritional supplementation should be defined as the process of making a person's diet complete in all six basic nutrients, according to the recommended daily allowances, through the addition of other food items. The dietitian in a cancer hospital quickly learns that a maintenance diet for a cancer patient requires supplementation beyond the idealistic RDA's. The cancer patient is often malnourished at presentation, taking catabolic drugs, and/or in a hypermetabolic state due to treatment or disease. The goal of the dietitian is to have the patient ingesting a normal, well-balanced diet at the end of the hospital stay or therapy. However, this "normal" state is usually inclusive of various dietary supplements if the patient is in need of weight gain or unable to tolerate large amounts of food.

INDICATIONS FOR NUTRITIONAL SUPPLEMENTATION

At M. D. Anderson Hospital, we utilize certain objective criteria in determining when nutritional supplementation is necessary. A typical candidate for supplementation has one or more of the following problems:

1. Weight loss of 5% or more
2. Evidence of malnutrition
3. Difficulty in assimilating nutrients
4. Mechanical difficulty managing food
5. Problems with food preparation
6. Treatment with aggressive gastrointestinal (GI)-toxic therapies without the benefit of intravenous hyperalimentation

The reasons for these problems are many and are responsible for altered intake, directly affecting the nutritional status of the cancer patient.

Many patients initially present with anorexia and cachexia due to their disease state or therapy. The mechanism responsible for the anorexia that occurs in cancer patients is not completely understood. It has been theorized to be metabolically activated or a result of other specific problems.

The treatment of the disease often predisposes patients to nutritional problems. Radiation therapy may cause impaired taste sensitivity, bowel damage, malabsorption, stenosis, obstruction, stomatitis, mucositis, and esophagitis. Surgical intervention may warrant preoperative and postoperative nutritional build-up for many patients, and certain types of surgery result in nutritional problems. Examples of this would be gastrectomies and intestinal resections that may cause malabsorption, decreased absorption of many nutrients, and vitamin deficiencies. Chemotherapy presents a variety of problems affecting food intake, the most common being nausea, vomiting, oral ulceration, mucositis, adynamic ileus, and diarrhea.

Taste abnormalities are common in this population and may be one of the factors contributing to anorexia and weight loss in the cancer patient. Several studies cite elevated taste thresholds for sweet and lowered thresholds for bitter (urea) (5). However, clinical observations at M. D. Anderson Hospital show lowered thresholds to both sweet and bitter. Patients with decreased bitter thresholds usually refuse beef, poultry, fish, and eggs but are able to tolerate cheese and milk products. Present literature theorizes that taste aversions may be related to the amino acid composition of ingested food in relationship to the imbalances in the patient's body (3,8).

Pain and nausea may also interfere with a patient's food in take. The administration of analgesics and antiemetics for relief at mealtime is often initiated by the medical team before nutritional supplementation can begin. Behavior modification may be attempted with patients exhibiting conditioned responses. Depression may contribute to decreased intake. Emotional support versus the use of psychopharmocological agents is recognized as the therapy of choice in this situation (4). These complex problems result in many patients requiring supplementation. Therefore, nutritional supplementation is indicated to increase weight and nutritional status, to meet increased nutrient needs during therapy, and to provide a concentrated source of nutrients for patients unable to eat enough.

TYPES OF NUTRITIONAL SUPPLEMENTS

There is a large variety of nutritional supplements available for inpatient and outpatient use. These products have been placed in two major groups: commercial, and low-cost, readily available supplements.

Commercial Supplements

The group of commercial supplements encompasses products ranging from nutritionally complete feedings to modular supplements (see Tables 1–4).

Nutritionally Complete Formulas

Nutritionally complete formulas include three basic types of feedings: intact protein, milk-containing products; intact protein, lactose-free formulas; and defined formula diets. Intact protein, milk-containing products are liquid supplements that provide

TABLE 1. Intact protein, milk-containing products

Product/100 cc	Sustacal	Sustagen plus Water	C.I.B. + Milk	Compleat-B	Formula 2	Nutri 1000
Protein (g)	6.0	10.4	5.8	4.3	3.8	4.0
Protein source	Casein soy isolate	Nonfat dry milk Ca caseinate	Milk, soy isolate nonfat dry milk Na caseinate	Beef casein	Nonfat dry milk, beef, casein, albumin	Skim milk
Fat (g)	2.3	1.6	3.1	4.3	4.0	5.5
Fat source	Soy oil	Milk fat	Milk fat	Corn oil, beef fat	Corn oil, beef fat, egg yolk	Corn oil
CHO (g)	13.8	29.6	13.5	12.8	12.3	10.1
CHO source	Corn syrup solids, sucrose, lactose	Corn syrup solids, sucrose, lactose, glucose	Corn syrup solids, sucrose, lactose	Maltodextrins, fruits, sucrose, vegetables, orange juice, lactose	Sucrose, lactose, dextrose, wheat flour, orange juice, vegetables	Dextrin-maltose, sucrose, lactose, dextrose
kcal/100 cc	100	173	120	107	100	106
Lactose (g)	1.67	8.6	NAPH	2.4	3.74	5.01
mOsm/kg H_2O	625	1,200	2,000	405–490	435–510	400
Na meq/mg	4.0/92.5	5.2/120	4.0/93.1	7.4/170	2.7/63	2.3/52.8
K meq/mg	5.3/205.6	8.1/315.6	7.0/273.5	3.6/140	4.9/191	3.8/147.8
Ca meq/mg	5.0/100	15.8/315.6	7.8/156.5	3.4/67	5.5/110	6.0/120.5
P meq/mg	5.9/91.7	15.2/235.6	9.8/148.5	9.8/150	6.1/95	6.1/95.1
Residue level	Low	Low	Low	Medium	Medium	Low

Volume needed to meet 100% RDA's for protein, vitamins, and minerals	1,080 cc	960 cc	1,373 cc	1,600 cc	2,000 cc	1,920 cc
Manufacturer	Mead Johnson	Mead Johnson	Carnation	Doyle	Cutter	Cutter
General comment	a, b	a, b	a	b	b, c	a, b

C.I.B., Carnation Instant Breakfast; NAPH, not available, presumed high. Composition data calculated from manufacturer's product information based on standard dilution vanilla flavored supplements used. From ref. 11.

[a] Recommended for oral feeding due to good patient acceptance.

[b] Recommended for tube feeding.

[c] Not recommended for oral feeding due to poor patient acceptance.

TABLE 2. *Intact protein, low lactose*

Product/100 cc	Ensure	Ensure Plus	Isocal	Osmolite
Protein (g)	3.7	5.5	3.4	3.7
Protein source	Casein, soy isolate	Na and Ca caseinate soy isolate	Casein soy isolate	Na and Ca caseinates soy isolate
Fat (g)	3.7	5.3	4.4	3.8
Fat source	Corn oil	Corn oil	Soy oil MCT oil	MCT oil, corn oil, soy oil
CHO (g)	14.5	19.7	13.0	14.3
CHO source	Corn syrup solids, sucrose	Corn syrup solids, sucrose	Corn syrup solids	Corn syrup solids (glucose polymers)
kcal/100 cc	100	150	100	106
Lactose (g)	0	0	0	0
mOsm/kg H$_2$O	450	600	350	300
Na meq/mg	3.2/74	4.6/106	2.3/52.1	2.4/54.2
K meq/mg	3.3/126.8	4.9/190	3.3/130	2.2/87.5
Ca meq/mg	2.6/52.8	3.2/63	3.1/62.5	2.7/54.2
P meq/mg	3.4/52.8	4.0/63	3.4/52.1	3.5/54.2
Residue level	Low	Low	Low	Low
Volume needed to meet 100% RDA's for protein, vitamins, and minerals	1,920 cc	1,920 cc	1,920 cc	2,000 cc
Manufacturer	Ross	Ross	Mead Johnson	Ross
General comment	a, b, c	b, c, d, e	b, d	b, d

Composition data calculated from manufacturers' product information. From ref. 11.

[a] Recommended for oral feeding due to good patient acceptance.
[b] Recommended for tube feeding due to good patient tolerance.
[c] Flavor packets available for increased palatability.
[d] Not recommended for oral feeding due to poor patient acceptance.
[e] Patient must be gradually increased to full strength tube feeding due to hypertonicity of solution.

complete nutritional maintenance. They are usually suitable for both oral and tube feedings, and average 1 kcal per cc. These supplements are indicated for use in the nutritional maintenance or build-up of patients with active digestion and no lactose intolerance. Examples of this type of supplement are: Sustacal, Formula II, Nutri-1000, and Meritene.

Intact protein, lactose-free formulas have been developed for complete nutritional maintenance of patients with inadequate lactase concentrations or those with secondary lactose intolerance induced from surgery, radiation, or disease. Examples of these products are: Ensure, Ensure Plus, Lolactene, and Isocal. These supplements may be used orally or as tube feedings.

Defined formula diets are virtually fiber-free, semisynthetic formulas that can serve as oral or tube feedings for patients with minimal digestive capability. These products may be used as complete diets or supplements. However, poor taste acceptance often makes tube feeding the preferred method of administration. At M. D. Anderson Hospital, tube feedings utilizing these products are normally administered by continuous drip method, beginning with half-strength solutions and advancing to full-strength. Many of these products are available with flavorings that increase palatability, making oral ingestion more acceptable. Several of these products can be mixed with gelatin, flavoring extracts (1), fruit juices, and carbonated beverages to increase patient acceptance. These feedings are low in residue, so they can be incorporated into clear-liquid diets. Indications for use are:

1. Management of patients with gastrointestinal disease requiring the lower digestive tract be placed at rest
2. Provision of total oral nutrition for patients prior to bowel surgery
3. Malabsorption
4. Jejunal feedings

Examples of defined formula diets are Flexical, Vivonex, and Precision L.R.

TABLE 3. Defined formula diets: products containing amino acids, hydrolyzed protein, or protein isolates

Product/100 cc	Flexical[a]	Vivonex[a]	Vivonex HN[a]	Precision HN[b]	Precision LR[b]	Precision Isot[c]	Vital[d]
Protein (g)	2.24	2.1	4.2	4.4	2.63	2.9	4.2
Protein source	Amino acids, casein hydrolysate	Amino acids	Amino acids	Egg albumin	Egg albumin	Egg albumin	Hydrolyzed soy whey and meat, free amino acids
Fat (g)	3.4	0.1	0.1	0.05	0.08	3.0	1.03
Fat source	Soy oil, MCT oil, soy lecithin	Safflower oil	Safflower oil	Soybean oil, mono- and diglycerides	Soybean oil, mono- and diglycerides	Soybean oil, mono- and diglycerides	Sunflower oil
CHO (g)	15.4	22.6	21.0	21.8	24.9	14.4	18.5
CHO source	Corn syrup solids, modified tapioca starch, citrate	Glucose oligo-saccharides	Glucose, glucose oligo-saccharides	Maltodextrins, sucrose	Maltodextrins, sucrose	Maltodextrins, sucrose, glucose oligo-saccharides	Glucose oligo-saccharides, polysaccharides
kcal/100 cc	100	100	100	100	110	100	100
Lactose (g)	0	0	0	0	0	0	0
mosmol/Kg H₂O	723	500	850	557	525	300	450
Na meq/mg	1.6/36	3.7/86	3.4/77	4.4/100	3.0/70	3.5/80	1.96/45
K meq/mg	3.2/124	3.0/117	1.8/70	2.3/90	2.2/87	2.5/96	3.5/137
Ca meq/mg	3.0/60	2.2/44	1.3/27	2.0/40	2.9/58	3.2/64	3.9/78.4
P meq/mg	3.2/50	2.9/44	1.7/27	2.6/40	3.7/58	4.1/64	5.0/78.4
Residue level	Low	Low	Low	Low	Low	Low	Low

Volume needed to meet 100% RDA's for protein, vitamins, and minerals	2,000 cc	1,800 cc	3,000 cc	2,850 cc	1,710 cc	1,560 cc	1,500 cc
Manufacturer	Mead Johnson	Eaton	Eaton	Doyle	Doyle	Doyle	Ross
General comment	e, f,	f, g	e, f	f, g	f, g	f, g	f, g

Composition data calculated from manufacturer's product information based on standard dilution.
From ref. 11.
[a] Unflavored product-flavors available.
[b] Citrus flavor.
[c] Vanilla flavor.
[d] Banana flavor.
[e] Not recommended for oral feeding due to poor patient acceptance.
[f] Recommended for tube feeding due to good patient tolerance.
[g] Recommended for oral feeding due to good patient acceptance.

TABLE 4. Supplements

Product/100 cc	Polycose	MCT oil	Pedialyte	Citrotein	Delmark eggnog	Controlyte	Sustagen and milk[a]	Sustaprotein
Protein (g)	0	0	0	4.0	6.0	Trace	5.6	30
Protein source	—	—	—	Egg albumin	Nonfat dry milk, egg albumin	—	Nonfat dry milk, Ca caseinate milk	82% hydrolyzed collagen[b] 18% free amino acids[b]
Fat (g)	0	93.3	0	0.17	3.6	9.6	3.8	0
Fat source	—	MCT oil	—	Mono- and diglycerides soybean oil	Cottonseed oil, soybean oil, egg yolk	Soybean oil	Milk fat	—
CHO (g)	50	0	5.0	12.0	14.8	28.6	10.4	0
CHO source	Modified corn starch	—	Dextrose	Maltodextrins, sucrose, glucose	Maltodextrins, lactose, sucrose	Maltodextrins	Sucrose, lactose, corn syrup solids, glucose	—
kcal/100 cc	200	775	20	65.3	116	200	98.2	120
Lactose (g)	0	0	0	0	NAPH	0	NAPH	0
mOsm/kg H_2O	570	NA	80	500	NA	570	NA	NA
Na meq/mg	2.7/62	0	3.0	2.9/68	4.0/91.6	0.26/6.0	3.2/74	Trace
K meq/mg	Does not exceed 1 meq (K, Ca, P)	0	2.0	1.7/68	6.7/262.5	0.08/3.2	5.2/203	Trace
Ca meq/mg		0	0.4	5.2/104	10.2/204	0.08/1.6	9.0/179	Trace
P meq/mg		0	0	6.7/104	10.5/162.5	0.10/1.6	9.0/139	Trace
Residue level	Low	Low	Low	Low	NA	Low	NA	Low
Type of supplement	Caloric supplement	Caloric supplement	Caloric and electrolyte supplement	Protein, mineral, and vitamin supplement	Protein and calorie supplement	High calorie-restricted protein restricted electrolyte supplement	Protein and calorie supplement	Liquid protein supplement
Manufacturer	Ross	Mead Johnson	Ross	Doyle	Delmark	Doyle	Mead Johnson	Mead Johnson

NA, not available; NAPH, not available, presumed high. Composition data calculated from manufacturer's product information based on standard dilution. From ref. 11. [a] Vanilla flavor used. [b] Protein quality consistent with ideal amino acid pattern.

Nutritionally-complete formulas have several advantages and disadvantages for the dietitian and patient. These products are convenient, require little to no preparation, and are easy to store, order, and administer.

Disadvantages of these nutritionally complete formulas lie mainly in their fixed composition. Patients with metabolic imbalances are often unable to tolerate one or more of the nutrients in the formula when given in the volume necessary to meet all nutrient requirements (11). Therefore, to meet the needs of a majority of patients, several different types of supplements must be stocked (2). Other disadvantages of these supplements are cost and lack of variety.

Modular Feeding

The concept of modular feedings arose chiefly from the necessity to reduce the stock of nutritional supplements, yet still meet individualized patient needs. Feeding modules consist of one basic nutrient: protein, fat, or carbohydrate. These modules can be combined and, with the addition of vitamins and minerals, form a complete feeding (2).

Anorexia in the cancer patient makes it necessary that a supplement contain the highest concentration of nutrients in the smallest volume, yet still be palatable. Feeding modules provide the dietitian with the ability to concentrate the most needed nutrients in a small volume without having to depend upon the patient to ingest large volumes of standardized formulas. These modules can be added to other standardized supplements or food items to concentrate the nutrient density of the food. Modular protein components serve as helpful adjuncts to diet therapy in a cancer population, since aversions to protein-rich foods are common.

Modular feedings do have the disadvantage of requiring individualized preparation. Since these modules must be mixed together, there may be lack of consistency in composition and quality.

Low Cost, Easily Available Supplements

Low-cost, easily available supplements are food products that can be purchased at a local grocery store by the patient. Taken alone, or when mixed with other ingredients, these foods form a high-calorie, high-protein product for supplementation of the patient's diet. Since the definition of nutritional supplementation includes any food item that adds missing nutrients to the diet, cheese, peanuts, peanut butter, and milk would also be considered under this heading. Other examples of low-cost supplements are: Instant Breakfast, Granola Bars, Space-Sticks, Breakfast Bars, eggnogs, milkshakes, high-protein milk made with the addition of powdered milk, and pureed tube feedings. Patients are often given copies of supplementary drink, tube feeding, or liquid diet recipes for home use. These recipes can all be made with typical household food items.

Advantages of using this type of product are multiple. There is decreased cost to the patient, the patient has the ability to vary the supplement as desired, and the patient and family can become more involved in his nutrition care plan. A disadvantage of these supplements is that they require preparation, so the patient and family must have the facilities and time necessary to make them.

It is important to know what a patient's living situation and finances will be outside the hospital in order to determine which type of supplement is best suited for his needs.

CRITERIA FOR PRODUCT SELECTION

Nutrient Quality

In choosing a supplement for use in an institution or with a particular patient, the quality of the product must be examined. Obviously, one must be certain the supplements being recommended or provided for use are of high quality, prior to determining which best suits a patient's needs. Quality comparison of products should be based upon protein form and quality, and carbohydrate and fat sources and amounts. Other factors to be considered are the addition of vitamins and minerals to the products.

Protein

Recently, there has been information reporting that absorption of certain dipeptides and tripeptides may be more efficiently utilized than free amino acids in normal volunteers (10). However, these findings do not agree with studies done on patients with short-bowel syndrome (13). There is not yet sufficient data available on the use of peptides in malabsorption states to warrant a blanket recommendation for their use over free amino acids or other forms of protein. There are improved taste, patient acceptance, and cost differences between whole protein, hydrolysates, and amino acids that would make the use of whole protein the preferred choice except in cases where malabsorption is evident (2). Since the degree of maldigestion differs greatly among patients, the form of the protein may not be as important to tolerance as the manner in which it is administered (12).

Animal proteins are considered to be of the highest quality since they have high digestibility and all essential amino acids are available. Plant proteins tend to be lower quality proteins since they are often limited in one or more amino acids and have poor digestibility. To provide essential amino acids at levels comparable to animal protein, plant proteins must be ingested in much larger quantities, eaten in combination with complementary protein sources, or supplemented with the limiting amino acid (6).

Fortunately, most commercially available, nutritionally complete products utilize proteins of high biological value. The determining factor in choosing between these supplements may become cost per gram of protein, since protein is the most costly and critical ingredient of a formula (6). In comparing protein modules, protein quality must be scrutinized. This is especially true of the liquid protein supplements and protein tablets that have recently flooded the market.

Carbohydrate

Carbohydrate is generally the major source of calories in a nutritionally complete supplement. The carbohydrate source is important for two major reasons:

Lactose Intolerance

The addition or deletion of milk in supplements may be a critical reason for choosing one product over another (2). Many cancer patients requiring nutritional support have an intolerance to lactose secondary to treatment or due to lactase deficiency.

Osmolality

Carbohydrate is also a major factor affecting the osmolality of a formula. Starches, dextrins, and glucose oligosaccharides are less osmotically active than mono- or disaccharidases (2,12). Oligosaccharides and longer-chain carbohydrates are not sweet, so they may be included in large amounts for caloric purposes, with the addition of sucrose or glucose for increased palatability (12).

Fat

Fat is the most difficult nutrient to digest, therefore, its digestion and absorption is commonly impaired in cancer patients. The presence of fat in levels above those necessary to prevent essential fatty acid deficiency should be considered in choosing a formula for patients known to have impaired digestion or absorption. Formulas low in fat, or those that incorporate medium chain triglycerides (MCT), may be useful in this patient population (12). MCT may preferentially be used as a fat source since it is easily metabolized. Caution is urged when using MCT in patients who have a tendency toward hepatic encephalopathy. The provision of large amounts of MCT to patients also should be monitored, since the absorption of large quantities has been associated with increased ketone bodies and acidosis (12).

Patients not exhibiting problems with digestion and absorption may benefit from formulas containing a higher fat content. Fat contributes calories without increasing the osmolality of the formula. Higher fat content also adds palatability and satiety value. Formulas containing about 20% of the calories from fat have been suggested to be ideal for palatability without causing rapid filling (9).

Minerals and Vitamins

Most commercial formula diets are nutritionally complete, containing all minerals and vitamins in amounts which meet the National Research Council's recommended daily allowances. This level may be adequate for many patients. However, patients who are severely malnourished may require additional vitamin and mineral supplements. Vitamins and minerals in formulas may, however, necessitate the use of different nutritional supplements if the patient has metabolic problems requiring certain mineral or vitamin deletions from his diet.

Nutritional Assessment

After evaluating the quality of supplementary products available for use, it is necessary to determine which ones are advisable for use with a particular patient. The patient's nutritional status should be assessed by methods previously discussed in this book. Knowledge of the patient's medical history is important for determining whether there are any medical contraindications for the use of specific supplements. The most needed nutrient, the most limited nutrient, the cost of the supplement, or a combination of these factors may be the basis for deciding which supplements will be offered to the patient.

The amount of supplement necessary for each patient is highly variable, depending upon the patient's basal energy expenditure, activity level, and whether weight maintenance or weight gain is necessary. The true metabolic needs for the cancer patient are not known, but since there is host-tumor competition for nutrients, the patient should be considered to be in a hypermetabolic state. The nutritional status of the patient who is septic is probably a close analogy, since the cancer patient and the septic patient require increased calories.

The Harris-Benedict equation is the preferred method for calculating basal energy expenditure (BEE) since it takes into account height, age, weight, and sex rather than weight alone (kcal/kg). The equation is as follows:

Men: BEE $= 66 + (13.7 \times$ wt in kg$)$
$+ (5 \times$ ht in cm$) - (6.8 \times$ age in yr$)$
Women: BEE $= 655 + (9.6 \times$ wt in kg$)$
$+ (1.7 \times$ ht in cm$) - (4.7 \times$ age in yr$)$

Blackburn (2) states that the patient in a catabolic state can be placed in positive nitrogen balance by routinely providing oral intakes of $1.54 \times$ BEE for 24 hr. Once the caloric needs for a patient are established, calories not being routinely provided by the patient's present diet should be ingested in the form of supplements.

Approximately 16% of caloric expenditure during stress comes from protein sources; therefore, Blackburn (2) recommends that 16% of the calculated caloric needs be from protein intake. The rest of the calories should be from nonprotein sources, to attain a 1:150 nitrogen to calorie ratio.

Patient Acceptance and Tolerance

Once the type and amount of supplement has been decided upon, the work of the dietitian is only half over. The final evaluation of the nutritional supplement lies with the patient. Obviously, if a patient finds the flavor offensive, he will not take a supplement regardless of how well it fulfills his needs. The cancer patient is known to have taste aversions and decreased taste acuity. Many supplements that are not routinely accepted for oral use by the general hospital patient may be well tolerated by a cancer patient. Conversely, nutritional supplements that are well tolerated by most patients may be rejected by the cancer patient. It is wise not to discount the use of any supplement because its flavor is unacceptable to the dietitian or staff.

Experience has proven that when patients are given active roles in supplementation, their acceptance increases. This can be accomplished by several methods:

1. Ask patients if they have been using any special supplement at home. If so, try to duplicate it.

2. Test trays consisting of small amounts of several appropriate supplements may be given to patients for sampling. They can then choose which formulas and flavors they prefer, and determine when they will receive them.

3. Patients may be given nutrient modules to be kept in their rooms, and instructed to use these supplements in foods not provided by the dietary department.

Flavor fatigue may become a problem after a supplementation program has been instituted; thus, close monitoring of the patient's intake is needed. The patient is encouraged to use different supplements, or the same supplement in a different form at each meal or nourishment time. Exotic flavors of supplements are not usually tolerated for long periods, but may provide a necessary change of pace for a long-term patient. This "exotic" flavoring may be created with the addition of flavoring extracts or fruit juices (1).

If the patient is unable to consume large amounts of food, initiation of a supplementation program should begin in small increments. Four ounces of liquid supplement is often all a patient can tolerate and still eat three meals a day.

Patients often refuse to participate in their supplementation programs. Patients who have been suffering from nausea and vomiting may not be willing to try something new. Also, many patients cannot be convinced of the importance of nutrition, so other steps must be taken to assure nutritional adequacy in their diets.

In the eyes of the patient, the attending physician has more credibility than any other health team member. Reinforcement by the physician of the importance of nutrition and the consumption of diet supplements often makes the patient more willing to accept supplemental feedings.

Supplementation can be initiated as meal replacement. This means that liquid supplements may be given orally or by tube as the major source of calories, with regular food taken as between-meal nourishments. As the patient's intake of solid food increases, the amount of meal replacement is gradually decreased (7).

Administration of supplements as medication may be necessary for the patient who will not accept food supplements, or does not take them regularly. These supplements are given by nurses as prescribed by physicians. Nursing staff routinely charts administration of medicines, so this method also provides a means of assessing the patient's intake without a calorie count. If the patient still refuses supplementation, then tube-feeding should be initiated for nutritional maintenance.

Patient Tolerance

Patient tolerance is the final step in product selection. It is essential that a supplementation program be started at least one day prior to therapy for the patient to determine his tolerance to the feedings. Patients started on new supplements immediately before GI-toxic therapy may attribute side-effects of therapy to the supplements. Side-effects from previous therapy must be noted before initiating supplementation to determine if side-effects are preexisting conditions or due to the supplement.

Tolerance is of great importance in tube feedings. Lactose intolerance may initially be seen when large amounts of milk-based formula are given by tube. If the patient accepts and tolerates the feedings, then the supplementation plan is ready to be initiated.

THE ROLE OF THE DIETITIAN

The role of the dietitian is basically divided into three areas: psychological support, product selection, and education.

Psychological Support

One must realize that the cancer patient has an underlying fear of death throughout treatment. The wasting away of his body and the loss of his hair are significant reminders of the disease. Therefore, the patient often views nutrition and the building-up of his body as a major role in the battle against cancer. Patients will often have the philosophy that looking healthy means that they are healthy. Dietitians at M. D. Anderson Hospital encourage patients to build themselves up nutritionally to tolerate their therapies better. One should avoid conveying the idea that good nutrition by itself will prevent the disease from taking its toll.

One major idea that is stressed is that nutrition is the one area of the patient's treatment that he and his family can control. Treatment, hospitalization, and tests are controlled by the health care team, and the patient is given little choice. The ability to take an active role in some aspect of his treatment thus becomes quite beneficial to the independent patient. Families often feel helpless, almost outsiders during the patient's treatment, whereas the family can play an important role in the nutritional care of the patient through encouragement of food intake and suggestions of favorite foods. The family is especially important in the outpatient setting, since they may be chiefly responsible for food and supplement preparation or the actual feeding of the patient by mouth or tube.

Product Selection

The dietitian is the expert on nutritional formulas available for use. She may take a passive or an active role in the supplementation of patients. The dietitian can wait for orders from the physician to begin supplementation, or she can initiate supplementation for patients as she deems necessary. The dietitian may accept the product chosen by the physician for supplementation, or after conferring with the patient for tolerance and taste preferences, she may suggest a change to a product that better suits the purpose and the patient.

Although physicians are becoming increasingly aware of the importance of nutrition in the cancer patient, they do not always consider it before treatment, tumor response, and infection. It is the primary role of the dietitian to consider nutrition as an important adjuvant therapy, and use this knowledge of products, tolerance, and preferences to benefit the patient.

Education

The dietitians at M. D. Anderson Hospital serve to educate patients, families, nursing staff, and physicians regarding nutritional supplementation. Taste panels are routinely conducted for the medical staff to acquaint them with available supplements and their indications for use. Handbooks on nutritional supplements have been compiled for use by the physician and dietitian and are given to medical staff at this time. Taste panels are also held for patients and family members. This has been found to be a useful tool for initiating further communication regarding the nutritional support of the patient. Educational materials developed by staff or pharmaceutical companies are given to patients and families at this time and/or at discharge. Dietitians also try to inform patients where commercial supplements may be purchased and make known to them the various community services available to the cancer patient if funds are needed for special equipment for feeding purposes.

In summary, nutritional supplementation of the cancer patient is one of the major and most challenging roles the dietitian plays. It is important that all health care members in and out of the hospital be aware of the preventability and reversibility of malnutrition in this population. It behooves the dietitian to be knowledgeable of the various products available and their indications, and to be aggressive in their use. It is through this continued interest and action that nutrition will become a primary adjuvant therapy in the treatment of cancer.

REFERENCES

1. Behl, C. R., Agarawala, B. P., Guidici, R. A., and Galinsky, A. M. (1976): Improved taste acceptability for an oral hyperalimentation dosage form. *Am. J. Hosp. Pharm.,* 33:1014–1017.
2. Blackburn, G. L., and Bistrian, B. R. (1976): Nutritional care of the injured and/or septic patient. *Surg. Clin. North Am.,* 56:1195–1224.
3. DeWys, W. D. (1977): Anorexia in the cancer patient. *Cancer Res.,* 37:2354–2358.
4. DeWys, W. D., and Herbst, S. H. (1977): Oral feeding in the nutritional management of the cancer patient. *Cancer Res.,* 37:2429–2431.
5. DeWys, W. D., and Walters, K. (1975): Abnormalities of taste sensation in cancer patients. *Cancer,* 36:1888–1896.
6. Doyle Pharmaceutical Company (1976): Evaluation of protein quality.
7. Hoover, C. J., Maini, B. S., Bistrian, B. R., Schlamm, H. T., Wade, J. E., and Blackburn, G. L.: Use of a defined formula diet to prevent malnutrition in patients with advanced cancer. *JPEN, (in press).*
8. Keusch, G. T. (1977): Impact of nutrition on nutritional status: Resume of the opening discussion. *Am. J. Clin. Nutr.,* 30:1233–1235.
9. McCamman, S., Beyer, P. L., and Rhodes, J. B. (1977): A comparison of three defined formula diets in normal volunteers. *Am. J. Clin. Nutr.,* 30:1655–1660.
10. Mead Johnson Laboratories (1974): Liquid diets. *Perspectives in Nutrition,* No. 3.

11. Selig, D. E. (1978): *Nutritional supplementation at M. D. Anderson Hospital and Tumor Institute.* University of Texas Press.
12. Shils, M. E., Block, A. S., and Chernoff, R. (1976): Liquid formulas for oral and tube-feeding. *Clin. Bull.,* 6:151–158.
13. Sinko, V., and Linscheer, W. G. (1976): Absorption of different elemental diets in a short-bowel syndrome lasting 15 years. *Am. J. Dig. Dis.* 21:419–425.

Subject Index

Acetic acid, in lactose malabsorption, 112, 115
Adenosine triphosphate (ATP), 3-5
Adhesions, following ileostomy, 103
Adrenocorticosteroids, in chemotherapy, 70-72
Alanine, in extensive cancer, 6
Albumin
    drugs bound to, 13-14
    serum, as indicator of visceral protein status, 34-35, 136-137
Alimentary tract
    obstruction of, in cancer patients, 1, 180
    role in regulating food intake, 86
Alkylating agents, 71-72
Amino acids
    and food intake, 88-89
    synthetic, in elemental diets, 141
    utilization in extensive cancer, 6
Ampicillin, taken on empty stomach, 17
Anorexia
    in cancer patients, 1, 8, 83-94, 180
    in children, 132, 170
    emotional causes underlying, 91-94
    following chemotherapy, 76-77
Anthropometric measurement of nutritional status, 21, 23-25, 27-34, 136
Antibiotics, 16, 70-72
Anticonvulsants, and nutritional status, 15, 16
Antimetabolite agents, 71, 75
Antimicrobials, and nutritional status, 15, 16
Appetite
    loss, following radiotherapy, 50, 168, 170, 180
    suppression by drugs, 15
Arm muscle circumference (AMC), determination of, 32-34, 136

Basal energy expenditure (BEE), calculation of, 194
Basic metabolic rate, in cancer patients, 6
Behavior modification, in nutritional rehabilitation of cancer patient, 167-177
Beverages, high-calorie, following radiotherapy, 28
Bile salts, absorption of, 104
Body frame type, determination of, 28
Bone marrow transplantation, 122-125
Breast cancer, 65-66
Breath hydrogen analysis, 115

Cachexia, in cancer patient, 1, 6-7, 83-94, 180

Calories
    intake of, in children, 132-135
    in leukemia patient, 128
Carbohydrate, in nutritional supplements, 192
Cardiovascular overload, complication of IVH, 153
Central nervous system, tumors of, in children, 131
Chemotherapy
    in children, 132
    and diet, 13
    in leukemia patients, 122, 123
    and nutritional management, 69-81
    side effects of, 1, 73-74
Chest circumference, measurement of, in children, 136
Chlorpromazine, 16-17, 133
Cholecystitis, following ileostomy, 104
Cholelithiasis, following ileostomy, 104
Cloxacillin, taken on empty stomach, 17
Colostomy, nutritional management following, 105-109
Constipation
    following chemotherapy, 75
    following colostomy, 106-107
Corticosteroids, and nutritional status, 15, 16, 88
"Crabtree effect," 4-5
Creatinine height index (CHI), 37-38, 136-137
Crohn's disease, 99
Cytoxic agents, and nutritional status, 15, 16

Defined formula diet, 141-154, 181-188;
    see also Enteral elemental nutrition; Nutritional supplementation; Parenteral elemental nutrition
Dehydration, 58
Diarrhea
    in children, 132
    complication of enteral elemental nutrition, 147
    following abdominal irradiation, 53-55
    following chemotherapy, 75
    following colostomy, 107
    following ileostomy, 101, 104
Diet
    elemental, 141-154
    guidelines for ostomy patients, 107-109
    liquid, supplementation of, 59, 160-161
    progression following tube feeding, 164
Dietitian
    in care of patient with leukemia, 127-128
    in care of patient with malabsorption, 116